Thorsons Introdu...
HYPNOTI...

TELEPEN

This boo...   of ...

Thorsons Introductory Guide to HYPNOTHERAPY

Hellmut W. A. Karle,
BA, ABPsS, C Psychol, MBSECH

Formerly Principal Psychologist,
Guy's Hospital, London

Thorsons
An Imprint of HarperCollinsPublishers

Thorsons
An Imprint of HarperCollins*Publishers*
77–85 Fulham Palace Road,
Hammersmith, London W6 8JB

Published by Thorsons 1992
First published as *Hypnosis and Hypnotherapy:
A Patient's Guide* 1988
1 3 5 7 9 10 8 6 4 2

A catalogue record for this book
is available from the British Library

ISBN 0 7225 2535 4

Printed in Great Britain by
HarperCollinsManufacturing Glasgow

Dedication

To my parents

Acknowledgements

First and foremost thanks are due to Jennie Boys, who did as much work in revising and improving my draft as I did in writing it, if not even more.

Secondly, my thanks go also to Dr Ann Harvey, whose helpful suggestions were very welcome and useful.

Contents

Introduction

For some years now, interest in treatments for illnesses of all kinds outside the world of conventional western medicine, has been growing. At the same time as medicine and surgery are making tremendous and astonishing advances in saving life and in treating diseases and disorders of both the body and the mind, people are turning more and more to models of therapy that often derive from ancient practices, such as herbalism and acupuncture, or that seem somehow more in tune with the natural healing powers of the body, such as homoeopathy.

Hypnosis is increasingly in the public eye in this context. Not only are more and more doctors, dentists and psychologists using it as an additional technique within their own professional skills, but others, often lacking in any professional training or qualifications, advertise their services as 'hypnotherapists'.

In this book, I have tried to give an account of modern techniques of hypnotherapy and how they may be used to help many different kinds of problems, whether these show themselves in physical illnesses, pain etc., or whether they manifest themselves in psychological forms.

Chapter 1 gives a brief account of the history of hypnosis. In Chapter 2, I have tried to dispel some of the myths and misconceptions that are commonly believed, and to summarize contemporary theories and practices. In Chapter 3, the conditions for which hypnotic techniques are currently used are described, while Chapter 4 gives an account of how such techniques work.

Chapters 5 and 6 are intended as a guide to what to expect if thinking of having such treatment. In Chapter 7, advice is given on how to find where you may be able to get this kind of help. Chapter 8 summarizes the value of hypnosis both for the treatment of disorders and to improve the quality of life.

In the early 1960s, when I began using hypnosis in my work as a Clinical and Educational Psychologist, a book such as this would not have been published. At that time, those of my colleagues who used such techniques faced laughter, disbelief and sometimes suspicion. I experienced this myself then, but over the last twenty-five years, the situation has changed quite dramatically. Nowadays I am called on by surgeons and physicians at the hospital where I work to assist them in the treatment of their patients, as well as receiving requests from General Practitioners for help through hypnotic methods. Sometimes the pleas for help cannot be met: hypnosis is no panacea, nor has it magical powers, but it is achieving a useful role within the world of medicine and surgery, as well as in the fields of psychology and psychiatry. There are still relatively few doctors and psychologists who are trained and experienced in its use, but more and more are equipping themselves through specialized training. Over the next few years, hypnotherapy will become more widely available. At the same time, research and experiment are likely to improve the methods we use today as much as our present-day techniques have improved on those of the nineteenth century.

Chapter 1

History

The word for 'hypnosis' was invented only in the last century, but the method has existed for very much longer, probably as long as man himself. Magic, voodoo, shamanism, faith healing, yoga and all kinds of religious and primitive medical practices share many of the characteristics of what we now know as hypnosis and hypnotherapy. From time to time over the last two centuries or so, various people have developed techniques, sometimes genuine and helpful, at other times sheer fraud, that have depended on hypnosis. Much more commonly, hypnotic methods have been used without any kind of ceremony or ritual by ordinary people who never thought of themselves as using such techniques.

In 1794 a small boy developed a tumour that the doctor decided would have to be removed. This was long before the days of anaesthetics, so his mother sat beside him and told him a story that was so interesting that he hardly noticed what the doctor was doing. When the tumour had been cut away, and the whole operation was finished, he said he had felt no pain at all. Many years later, a book was published containing the story the little boy was told. The name of the author was Jacob Grimm, and the story was *Snow White*.

In the eighteenth century, interest in a variety of new healing methods was as lively as it is today. An Austrian doctor, Franz Anton Mesmer, found that he was able to cure people of different diseases without medicines or surgery. He came to believe that diseases were the result of blockages in, or disruption of, the flow of some kind of magnetic force in the

human body, and that using magnets could improve the flow of
the 'magnetic fluid' and so produce cures. He thought that all
kinds of things could be 'magnetized', and that contact with
such objects would transmit the curative power of magnetism
to patients and so relieve their illnesses. There are reports, for
instance, that he 'magnetized' a tree and that people who linked
themselves to this tree with ribbons or cords were thereby cured
of various diseases. He also developed a strange ritual in which
patients, usually in large groups, were arranged around a large
tub containing water, glass bottles and iron filings. Out of this
tub protruded iron bars which the patients held. In these
healing sessions, patients did indeed often get better,
sometimes quite dramatically, many of them having violent
seizures as soon as they came in contact with the iron bars. Very
similar things happened with the 'magnetized' tree: some
patients reacted quite violently, while others seemed to fall into
a deep sleep. Both in his *salon* and out of doors around a
'magnetized' tree, people seemed to be healed of all kinds of
illnesses.

Naturally, Mesmer became very famous in the Paris of his
time. He was unable, however, to obtain recognition from La
Société Royale de Médecine, but the French government,
apparently at the suggestion of Marie Antoinette, offered him a
life pension and sufficient money to set up a clinic. The
government, however, insisted that Mesmer must allow the
clinic to be supervised by government representatives, and this
he refused. Controversy flourished, with miraculous cures
being claimed and denied in turn. In 1784, the French King
appointed a Commission to carry out a thorough investigation.
This consisted of five Members of l'Académie Française and
four doctors from the University Faculty of Medicine, Paris.
Interestingly, Benjamin Franklin, the American scientist and
statesman, was amongst them. This supposed 'animal
magnetism' was demonstrated to the Commission by a disciple
of Mesmer, and numerous experiments were carried out. The
final report of the Commission concluded that the supposed
effects of 'animal magnetism' and of the 'magnetic fluid'

stemmed entirely from imagination, and nothing else. Sadly, Mesmer and his followers had made their treatments so dramatic and even melodramatic, riddled with mystery and elaborate window-dressing of all kinds, that they themselves lost track of what they were really doing. The belief that it was some form of magnetism that effected the cures distracted their attention away from what was really happening. As a result, both this Commission and a Committee of La Société Royale de Médecine were blinded to the fact that sometimes remarkable changes did occur in patients who were 'treated' by this method.

What Mesmer did, without recognizing it himself, and without it being recognised by the investigators, was to create an hypnotic state in his patients, not only by the rituals and equipment used, with its strong suggestions of some kind of power, but also by the way he handled his patients. He obviously had a most impressive manner, and made strange gestures towards his patients, with either explicit or hidden suggestions that something dramatic and strange would happen to them. He often did not have to make open or explicit suggestions that they would be healed of whatever was wrong, but this suggestion was strongly present in the whole situation.

After the two official reports were published in 1784, condemning Mesmer's practices and theories as worthless, he fell out of fashion, and ceased to be a public figure. His techniques were, however, continued by others. His name, of course, remains with us as a common word: we speak of a bird mesmerized by a snake, and of a mesmeric trance when we are completely fascinated.

The commissions that investigated Mesmer's claims dismissed them as of no value and based on fantasy, if not even fraud. This affected medical opinion throughout the world. In fact, because they look only at the idea of 'animal magnetism' which Mesmer, as well as others, supported, and did not investigate the experiences of his patients, in the way that perhaps we would do nowadays, they missed the only important part of what he was doing, and put a blight on anything that could be linked with 'animal magnetism' for nearly two hundred years. Anyone who spoke on a subject remotely connected with 'animal magnetism' or 'magnetic fluid' was automatically branded as either a fool or a cheat, so research and the development of hypnotic techniques was delayed for a century or more.

The crucial point of methods such as this, was missed by the commission of 1784, and by other Committees of Enquiry that were set up at intervals to investigate claims of healing through methods which did not fit the medical theories of the time. This was very well expressed by a pupil of Mesmer, Charles d'Eslon, in a book he published in Paris in 1780. He wrote: 'If the medicine of imagination is best, why should we not practise the medicine of imagination?'. The experience of the Mesmerists at the hands of the Commission is, perhaps, not so different from the experiences of practitioners of alternative therapies at the hands of the conventional medical establishment of the 1980's.

In the middle of the nineteenth century, a Scottish doctor, James Braid, published a book on what he called *Neurhypnology, or the Study of Nervous Sleep*. He invented the word 'neur-hypnosis', and from this we have derived the word 'hypnosis'. He, too, experimented with magnets, but found that they achieved nothing. He did, however, show that it was possible for people to go into a strange sleep-like state in which they were able to lose many symptoms of illness or injury. Braid compared this state with the paralysis which some animals show when extremely frightened, as, for example, a rabbit when faced with a stoat, or a bird before a snake. He believed that this state of 'fascination' could be deliberately produced and that going into that state in some way healed injury or disease.

Braid was not accepted by the medical profession of his time, any more than was another Scottish doctor, John Elliotson, who practised surgery both in India and later in Britain, using hypnosis to enable his patients to lessen the pain caused by the operations they had to undergo. Despite his detailed and well-researched reports on hypnotic anaesthesia, he too was dismissed by his colleagues.

Throughout the second half of the nineteenth century, despite the scorn and laughter of the medical and scientific community, hypnosis was studied and taught by an increasing number of doctors, both in Britain and on the continent. In France, hypnotic phenomena were studied and practised extensively, and controversy between two main schools of thought developed and flourished for many years. These were the Medical Faculty of the Salpêtrière, Paris, under Professor Jean-Martin Charcot, and the Nancy School under Hippolyte-Marie Bernheim. Charcot carried out extensive work on the link between hysterical disorders and hypnotic states. Despite the hostility of the medical profession to anything that had any connections with the discounted idea of animal magnetism, Charcot presented a paper on the nature of hypnosis to the French Academy of Sciences in 1882. His theories on the nature of hypnosis were further investigated, and were found, some years later, to be inaccurate, but, as a result of his determination and courage, the subject gradually became more respectable in scientific circles for a time.

Other eminent medical scientists soon followed his example. Professor Hippolyte-Marie Bernheim, at the University of Nancy, took a less academic or scientific approach than Charcot. He was interested principally in the practical application of hypnosis as a therapy. He claimed that the results of his researches, published in 1884, showed that hypnotherapy worked through the power of suggestion, and his descriptions of treatment through hypnosis are not so very different from modern practices. His theories on how these treatments worked were, however, very different from what we know now, and have been discounted by the results of more recent research. None the less, he is remembered and honoured today in the title of the Institute for the Study of Clinical Hypnosis and Psychotherapy at the University of Padua, which was named after him.

During the last quarter of the nineteenth century, more and

more physicians on the continent became interested in hypnosis, particularly in its application in the treatment of mental illnesses. One of the best-known of them was Sigmund Freud. Having studied hypnosis in France, under Professor Charcot, and its use in the treatment of psychological disorders, he used the technique himself for a time, but gradually came to believe that it was of little real value and began to develop other techniques to take its place. Initially, he used hypnosis to enhance the effects of suggestions he would make to try and remove symptoms. Later, as he became more and more convinced that psychiatric symptoms often represented memories, feelings and inner conflicts of which the patient was not conscious, he began to use hypnosis to uncover and release such hidden traumatic memories and feelings. Although these methods often seemed to produce satisfactory improvement in the condition of patients, the effects were often short-lived and left no lasting benefit. In time, Freud concluded that hypnosis was not an appropriate mode of treatment, and conceived the technique of 'free association' as a means of gaining access to the unconscious memories, feelings and thoughts of his patients. In fact, as one can see in retrospect, the technique he developed (and for which he is best known today – psychoanalysis), is very closely akin to hypnosis as it is practised today, although very different from the hypnotic methods of his own time. The process of free association is characterized by much the same features that we see in hypnosis, and some writers have argued that in fact Freud began to use hypnosis in a modern way at the moment that he believed he had abandoned it.

Despite the scepticism or outright disbelief of many eminent people, the British Medical Association apppointed a committee to 'investigate the nature of the phenomena of hypnotism; its value as a therapeutic agent; and the propriety of using it.' This led to a report published in 1892. The Committee carried out experiments which satisfied them that hypnosis as such was real and that it could and did have physical effects which could be of benefit to some patients.

They concluded that it had real value in the control of pain, in inducing sleep and alleviating many ailments that did not stem from physical damage. They also stated that they believed it could be dangerous if 'carelessly used', that is, either in the absence of adequate medical knowledge, or through intentional abuse. Despite their acceptance of hypnotic techniques as a proper form of treatment for doctors to use, none of their recommendations appeared to have any effect. Hypnosis continued to be either ignored or laughed at by medical practitioners for many years, both in Britain and abroad.

Towards the end of the century, interest within the medical profession waned again in Europe. In America, however, a number of academics and physicians continued to study the topic. Boris Sidis published a number of books on hypnosis in the first two decades of the twentieth century, in which he advocated its use in uncovering the unconscious roots of some abnormal or undesirable behaviour and actions. He was probably the first writer to point out the hypnotic character of Freud's technique of free association. Only a few isolated individuals, however, took the topic seriously during this period.

At the beginning of the twentieth century, with these very few exceptions, hypnosis was to be found only in fiction, drama and on the stage. The medical profession considered it to be either fraudulent, or of no medical significance or value. It was generally believed that only people lacking in strength of will and character could be hypnotized and that no honest physician would bring himself so low as to use a technique which belonged to the province of rogues and tricksters.

However, the subject never actually went away and by the 1930s, interest on the part of scientists, especially medical, grew once more. Careful and systematic investigations were begun, both by academic scientists and by doctors in clinical practice. The first modern book on the subject, *Hypnotism and Suggestibility* by C. M. Hull, was the beginning of a flood of books that is still growing. For the first time, hypnotism came under real scientific scrutiny. Up till then, it had only been demonstrated, usually in rather dramatic or even melodramatic ways, and generally only in the treatment of illnesses, but with little real attempt to study it systematically. Since then, research and clinical studies have been carried out in university departments and hospitals throughout the world.

In 1955, a report from another committee appointed by the British Medical Association gave official approval to the use of hypnosis in treating both physical and psychological disorders. Three years later the American Medical Association followed suit. Both in Britain and in the USA, training in hypnotherapy has been officially recommended for doctors, although thirty years later it is still rare in Britain to find this recommendation carried out.

Despite official approval, extensive use of hypnosis by doctors and psychologists, and in spite of continual academic research in universities, we are still at an early stage in our understanding of the nature of hypnosis. There is no generally agreed understanding of how it works, how it enables physical as well as mental processes to be modified and even controlled, or really about what hypnosis *is*. Knowledge is growing rapidly, especially about what can be done with hypnosis in many practical ways, and acceptance of such techniques in medicine and surgery is increasing. More and more practitioners in GP surgeries, dental practices, hospitals and clinics of all kinds will use hypnosis, often together with other forms of treatment, but there is still considerable resistance in the professional establishment.

When I began using hypnosis in my own practice some twenty-five or more years ago, I was regarded as slightly odd, perhaps even cranky, and even nowadays I still meet with scepticism, suspicion, and downright disbelief, from some of my colleagues. Suspicion of hypnosis as something that had for many decades been considered deceitful or worse, remains. Amongst the general public, many of the old ideas and myths about hypnosis are still commonly believed, fostered by novels, films and stage performances. In addition, there is no public control over the use of hypnosis in Britain, or in some other countries. In many countries, however, the use of hypnosis is restricted to people such as registered medical or dental practitioners, and clinical psychologists. In Britain, however, anyone may advertise himself as a hypnotherapist and 'treat patients', without any recognized medical or psychological training or qualifications. To be sure, the abuse of hypnosis in stage demonstrations has been limited by restricting such performances to clubs, by the Hypnotism Act of 1952, but in other countries such demonstrations have been outlawed altogether.

Because hypnosis is a powerful process, it has the potential for achieving important beneficial effects when properly used. Equally, however, simply because it *is* powerful, it is also dangerous in the wrong hands. Thus, since we unfortunately do not have any public or official control over its use, nor any recognized training for its professional use, in Britain, the public must be cautious in consulting hypnotists and choose carefully. The question of how to find a hypnotherapist who holds genuine qualifications and is a member of a valid profession, is discussed in Chapter 7.

Hypnosis is a powerful technique by which many different kinds of treatment can be undertaken. It gives additional power to many psychological and physical treatments. Its history is very chequered, and those that figure in it include honest and scientific persons as well as charlatans, frauds and tricksters. The situation today is different from, say, the last century, in that hypnosis is rapidly achieving respectability and respect, both in academic circles and in clinical practice. Rather as in past centuries, however, while there are many honest, skilled and ethical practitioners, there are also many who are less honest, less skilled and sometimes unethical.

Research continues, and new developments emerge all the time. National and international societies for the study and development of the practice of hypnotherapy flourish. Increasingly physicians, dentists, psychologists and others are being trained in the use of such methods and apply them in practice, not *in place of* other treatments, but to enhance the treatments already in use. As we learn more about what a human being is and how a human being works, so I believe we will use hypnosis more frequently, openly and explicitly, and, above all, more efficiently and effectively. The long and curious history of the subject has led to us developing a more scientific, objective, and reliable understanding of the whole process, but we still have a great deal to learn.

Chapter 2

What Hypnosis Is and What It Is Not

Most people when asked if they have ever been hypnotized answer 'No', and are nearly always mistaken. Almost everyone has at some time, perhaps even quite frequently, been in a hypnotic state without recognizing it. In childhood, day-dreaming which is so real to the child that the dream or imagined situation takes the place of ordinary reality, is essentially self-hypnosis. In adult life, many people still daydream occasionally, and most people will have episodes of absent-mindedness or abstraction at times, in which they are, as we say, 'in a world of their own'.

For instance, when driving down a familiar road you may suddenly realize that you have travelled several miles without being able to remember anything of that part of the journey. If you have a passenger at the time, he or she would be able to testify to the fact that during the period in which, apparently, you were 'not there', you drove perfectly competently, adjusting to road conditions, avoiding dogs and children, stopping at red lights and so on, and may even at the same time have been holding a perfectly coherent coversation. Yet, when you 'come to', you realize that you have no memory at all of the last few miles, and probably also that you cannot remember now what you were thinking about during that period. Or at another time you may be engrossed in something, watching a film on television, reading a book or absorbed in a hobby, when someone asks you a question, and you answer; perhaps they even hold a conversation with you. A little while later, however, when that conversation is mentioned again, you have absolutely no recollection of it.

In all these states, much the same thing has happened as happens in hypnosis. The consciousness of the individual concerned separates into two streams which are out of touch with each other. In hypnosis, as in the sort of abstracted states described earlier, these different lines or streams of thought and action become separated, so that you are actually aware of only one line of thought and action at a time, while the rest is being done on a sort of mental auto-pilot.

In everyday life, we can usually do two or even more things at once and be fully aware of all of them at the same time. For instance, frequently while driving, you can hold a conversation with a passenger and at the same time, perhaps, work out what you are going to say to the Bank Manager when you see him next day. You will be fully aware of that conversation, of your thoughts, and of what you are doing as a driver.

In a 'normal' frame of mind, there is a central line or stream of consciousness which acts to co-ordinate everything that is going on in your mind. This is rather like the conductor of an orchestra, directing which group of instruments is to be prominent and which should be in the background or even silent altogether. The conductor of your mind chooses at any particular moment which is to be central in your awareness and what is to be excluded. In an abstracted frame of mind, when you are daydreaming or wool gathering, or when you are in hypnosis, the conductor turns to a soloist and silences the rest of the orchestra. Then the soloist can be heard without distraction of any kind.

Another way of understanding what happens in such a state of abstraction, is to think of consciousness as a light, illuminating a room. Whatever is nearest the light is most brightly lit, and the rest of the room is rather dimmer. That is, whatever you are attending to especially, is uppermost in your consciousness, but you may be aware, rather less clearly, of many other things. Sometimes, when you are concentrating especially hard on some task or thought, the light becomes focused into a narrower beam, rather like a spotlight. As a result, whatever it is focused on is very brightly lit. Some light, however, still scatters around the room, so that everything else is dimly illuminated. In other words, in a state of strong concentration, you will be most vividly aware of the object of your attention, but at the same time, you may still be vaguely aware of everything else. In special states of abstraction, or in hypnosis, the light of your consciousness is even more precisely focused, and, rather like a laser beam, can be exclusively focused on a single point. Then no light at all will escape to the side, and the rest of the room will be in darkness. In that situation, you are conscious of the centre of your attention and of nothing else at all.

As a matter of plain fact, there is only one kind of hypnosis – *self hypnosis*. All hypnosis is self-induced, although a therapist, or various kinds of rituals, or incantations and the like, can help you to go into the hypnotic state more quickly or more easily. But only, and this must be emphasized, *only* if you go along with it and *choose* to go into the trance state will you do so.

It is generally claimed that no-one will act out of character in hypnosis, or will do anything in hypnosis to which they object. Sometimes people will point out that what they found themselves doing or saying in hypnosis did conflict with their moral or social standards, and that therefore, they would not have chosen to act or speak in that way. The point is that what we consciously believe and think of as our standards does not necessarily match up with the deeper levels of our personality. Sometimes (in fact, quite frequently), our more deeply hidden thoughts, feelings, and wishes can be very much in conflict with what we hold consciously, or what we want to believe about ourselves. In hypnosis, just as in dreams or under the pressure of great stress, we can find ourselves acting on the basis of these deeper and perhaps quite unconscious standards or feelings. When this happens in everyday life, we may say: 'I was beside myself' or 'I wasn't myself just then', but obviously, we *were* ourselves then, but acting from a much deeper and less conscious level than usually. The same is true of hypnosis. If secretly you would like to say or do things that in the ordinary way you would not allow yourself, then you may very well act out or say those things in hypnosis. In part this is, of course, because you feel, at a deep level, that being hypnotized somehow excuses you from responsibility or gives you permission to do or say these things. In part, however, it is also due to the fact that in hypnosis you can actually be free of the training and conditioning you received as a child; once again, you actually have *more* control than usually and so can do things that normally you would be *unable* to do because of your childhood training.

On the other hand, you will never do or say things in hypnosis which you find offensive or wrong at both deeper and more superficial levels. Nor will you ever do or say anything in hypnosis if you decide not to do or say these things. This is an essential aspect of the hypnotic state, one of its most important characteristics.

In hypnosis, you do not cease, as a rule, to be unaware or unconscious of what is going on around you. You may actually be aware of noises from outside the room, the tightness of your shoes, or any other stimulus, but your awareness of these things is somehow slightly distant or removed, as you are concentrating much more directly and completely on what the therapist is saying to you, and on what you are using the hypnosis for. It is only in the deepest hypnotic states, which we call 'somnambulistic' (which is very like sleep-walking), that you actually cease to be aware of anything except what is being suggested to you and the content of the hypnotic session. This is quite rare: probably only one person in ten can actually reach this depth of trance.

Another aspect of hypnosis is again something very familiar to almost everyone: that what you have in your thoughts or what you are picturing in your mind, affects your mood, your frame of mind, and your bodily sensations. For instance, most people when embarrassed, feel awkward and often find themselves blushing. Or if you concentrate your attention on a memory of an event that was very frightening or on the thought of something dangerous, you will feel yourself beginning to *feel* alarmed and even frightened, even though you may be sitting safely in your armchair at home. At the same time, you may find that your heart is beating faster than usual; you may go pale; feel your stomach going into knots; and you may even begin to sweat or go cold and clammy.

Any idea, thought or picture we hold in our minds will, if it has some emotional significance for us, produce the same reactions as if the event or situation were actually happening. In everyday life, we put up with such reactions, and try not to be too disturbed by them. Any disturbing memories that affect us in this way, we generally try to put out of our minds. For instance, when you find yourself getting more and more worried about something in your life – money, the state of your car, why your daughter is out so late, or whatever – you may switch on the television set or involve yourself in some task in order to distract yourself so that you can stop thinking about the worrying topic and so not feel the anxiety for a while. In contrast, we may dwell on pleasant memories and images for the sake of the good feelings they give us. Sexual fantasies or memories can affect us strongly, and we look forward to the prospect of something exciting or an enjoyable event, with pleasurable anticipation.

There is an old legend which illustrates that one's feelings can, and often do, have powerful effects. In the ancient city-state of Sparta, children were trained, from a very early age, to hide their feelings, and, especially, never to show pain. One day, a small boy on his way to school saw a fox-cub sitting at the side of the path. He stopped and played with the little animal for a time, and then realized he was going to be late for school. Quickly, he scooped up the cub, tucked it under his shirt and ran off to school. Sure enough, he was late, and, to punish him for being late, he was told to stand in the corner. He dared not say anything about the fox-cub, so held it against him as he stood quietly. After a little while, the cub became restless, so the little boy held on to it tighter. Bit by bit, the cub became more restless and tried to get free. It began to nip the boy with its teeth, but the boy hung on, not flinching, determined to be brave and strong. The cub began to bite, and still the boy held on. Gradually the cub began to bite more and more deeply, until, when the cub bit right through to his heart, the boy fell down, dead.

The same story is repeated almost daily in the experience of any doctor. Patients come with a pain in their abdomen, and investigations show that they have an ulcer eating away at the lining of their stomach. It is not just the acids of the stomach that are eating away at them, but the feelings which the patient has been hiding away, such as unacknowledged anger, resentment or disappointment, pretending they were not there or refusing to allow them open expression. These feelings have been nipping and chewing away at them, perhaps for years. What we hold in our hearts and minds is a part of our whole experience of being alive, and affects every part of our being, and will find expression in one way or another, through physical or psychological symptoms, or both. In this natural way, we may have no control over what happens, and may not even be aware or concious of what is going on, noticing only the outward symptons without understanding them, or their origins.

Hypnosis uses the same mechanisms as are involved in such experiences, but in contrast to what happens in everyday life, we can use these processes consciously, deliberately, purposefully and with control. For instance, a teenager was referred to me because she had become very unhappy, depressed and tense. I taught her how to go into the hypnotic state and then asked her to imagine herself on her favourite beach, enjoying the sunshine and the water. When we had finished she said to me: 'That's just the same as I've been doing on my own, when the other girls get at me so much that I can't stand it: I just go away inside myself and then it doesn't bother me so much'.

The way we think and what we think, affect the way we feel, and frequently we are strongly affected in our feelings and general or personal state by suggestions made by other people. If everyone you meet one day were to say to you: 'Oh dear, you do look unwell; shouldn't you be at home and in bed?', you would soon feel pretty ill and want to retire to bed! On the other hand, if you were to be greeted wherever you went with compliments on your appearance, your manner, and remarks on how well you are looking, you would soon feel pretty good, even if the day had started badly. The same idea is used in hypnotherapy: what you are thinking of yourself affects the way you feel and consequently the way you deal with life. However, your deepest and most important feelings about yourself may be quite different from and at odds with what you *think* you feel. When you become able to change what you hold in the deeper levels of your mind about yourself, then you are beginning also to take control of your life. In normal waking life, we can be quite strongly affected by suggestion. In hypnosis, this is even more the case, and one of the characteristics of the hypnotic state is that of increased susceptibility or greater openness to suggestion. In everyday life, suggestions made to us by other people, or by some part of our own minds, will affect us, often without our even being aware of it happening.

Quite a few years ago, I was teaching at a Summer School, and in the evening, after dinner, all the tutors went to a local inn for a few drinks before bed. I happened to be sitting by an open window, and laid my pipe on the sill to cool. When I reached for it later, I knocked it and it fell outside. One of the other tutors waved me back into my seat and insisted on fetching it himself. During the remainder of the evening, I felt somehow not quite one of the group, and only later realized that I had begun to feel much older than the rest of the group. Although I *was* a few years older than the others, I had begun to feel *much* older when treated as a senior. The implied suggestion had acted very powerfully on me.

In hypnosis, we make or accept suggestions consciously and deliberately, and so can use them to achieve something that we want, or something that will benefit us, and somehow that acceptance goes even deeper than it would in non-hypnotic states.

Hypnosis is all about control, but – unlike in fiction and

drama – real-life hypnosis is about *your own control* of yourself, your mind and body, and not at all about coming under the control of another person. In fiction, the usual belief is that the hypnotist takes over control and can make the subject, or rather the victim, do whatever he, the hypnotist, wants. Life as a hypnotherapist would be a lot easier if this were true (as we could then effect dramatic cures very quickly), but it is simply nonsense. Hypnosis allows you to control aspects of your whole being that normally you have no direct control over, but, and this is very important, it is always *your* control.

A story is told of Sigmund Freud from the days when he used hypnosis and taught others about it. I cannot guarantee that the story is actually true, but it describes accurately what would happen in such a situation. Dr Freud was demonstrating hypnosis to a group of students. He carried out an induction on a young woman (that is, he led her into a hypnotic trance state), and was about to carry out some experiments to show what could be done with hypnosis, when he was called out of the room. He handed over to his assistant, who began to make various suggestions to the woman which would demonstrate the fact that she was hypnotized. Having satisfied himself and the audience by various experiments that the woman was really in a hypnotic trance, he became rather less ethical. He made the suggestion that she should believe she was at home and that it was evening. That, as far as the patient was concerned, was fine. He suggested that she now wished to go to bed. That was fine too. But when he suggested that she was about to undress to take a bath she opened her eyes, slapped his face, and marched indignantly off the stage.

You can be hypnotized only if and when you agree to it. You stay in the trance only as long as you want to, and accept and act on only those suggestions that feel right to you. As I said before, there is only one person in the world that can hypnotize you, and that is you yourself. All that the hypnotist *can* do is to show you how to do it and lead the way. Nothing can happen in hypnosis that you do not agree to, and you simply cannot be made to do, think, or feel, anything you do not want to. That is really quite obvious since you and only you are in charge.

One point people sometimes raise about this needs clarification. If you watch, or perhaps take part in a demonstration of hypnosis at a nightclub or a party, you might very well think that these statements cannot be true, because you will see other people doing, or find yourself doing, all sorts of silly and embarrassing things, things you 'would not been seen dead doing'. At a party or in a club, with a few drinks inside you, and with your friends egging you on, you would be quite likely to do silly or even humiliating things quite willingly, even without hypnosis. Because of the situation, and because you, and the audience, *believe* that the hypnotist can make you do things, you go along with whatever he suggests. If the hypnotist is skilled and intelligent, he will not suggest anything that you would find really offensive, because if he did, it would not work and you would come out of the trance. He will suggest only the sort of things the person is likely to expect and accept, and so, as far as the audience is concerned, it works.

I hope that I have now made it clear that there is nothing magical about hypnosis, nothing occult or strange. It is an everyday experience, and when used for healing, it is the application of a natural talent that most people have to some extent, although, of course, some more than others. There is nothing alarming about it. On the contrary, it is one of the most relaxing, pleasant and comfortable experiences you can have. It does not involve losing or giving up control. The experience is under your control, and only yours, and the process can teach you a degree of control over your own mind and body that is not there for most of us in the ordinary waking state.

There are other characteristics of the hypnotic state that are also important to its use in therapy. While in hypnosis, the mind is partially freed from its dependence on external reality and normal logic. In dreams (which are closely related to hypnosis), totally illogical and unrealistic events seem thoroughly normal and possible, and the mind seems to be able to by-pass its normal reliance on things having to conform to everyday reality. In day-to-day life, when we see or hear something that does not make sense, we can dismiss it, ignore it, or change it in some way so that it does make sense. In hypnosis, we can accept what comes into our minds just as it comes, as in dreams, even if it does not obey what we believe to be the laws of nature. Dreams and hypnotic experiences can be rather like the verse which goes:

> He thought he saw a banker's clerk
> Descending from a bus.
> He looked again and saw it was
> A Hippopotamus.

> He thought he saw an elephant
> That played upon a fife.
> He looked again and saw it was
> A portrait of his wife.

For instance, if you are good at self-hypnosis and the idea is suggested to you that your right arm is beginning to feel lighter and lighter until it is as weightless as a balloon, you will find that your right arm starts to feel lighter and lighter and eventually, without any effort on your part, and if you 'let go' of that arm, it will gently float up into the air as though it really were as light as a balloon. You will feel quite definitely that you are not lifting your arm yourself, and that it is actually floating. Similarly, if you picture that you are putting one hand into a bowl of hot water, and that the hand is getting warmer as a result, the temperature of that hand will actually go up and your hand may go pink, just as it would in hot water. More practically, if you have a pain somewhere, and you accept the suggestion that the part where you feel the pain is going numb, you will actually find that the pain lessens and may disappear completely, as that part of your body goes numb.

In the wrong hands and in the wrong place, hypnosis can be wrongly used. As described earlier in the excitement, perhaps, of a party or a nightclub, with a few drinks inside you and your friends around you, you might volunteer for a stage show of hypnosis. If you do, you might very well end up making a complete fool of yourself, to the amusement of everyone in the party. You may also feel thoroughly ashamed afterwards. What is more, you might even not come out of the hypnotic state easily and comfortably and need professional help to overcome the effects of the experience. This is, of course, why some countries have made it a criminal offence to give such shows. In such a setting, some people are liable to get carried away by the mood of the party and end up doing things they would not agree to in other circumstances. I am quite sure none of my patients would do any of the silly things people do in the course of such shows, if I tried to get them to do them in my office. They would open their eyes, slap my face and walk out of my room. At a party, however, with the help of a little alcohol, I expect they could be persuaded to do all these things, and more – and would regret it afterwards.

Hypnosis can also be described as a state of intense concentration combined with total relaxation. In everyday life, if we become intensely interested in something, we tend to tense up physically. Think of a small child learning to write and working very hard at writing her name; almost certainly, the child's tongue will stick out and curl slightly with the effort of concentration. Or notice, when you are putting your whole mind to some task, that whatever parts of your body are not actively involved in the task in hand (your back, legs, hands or arms), may become quite rigid, so that when you stop doing whatever it was, you find you have to stretch because you have gone so stiff. On the other hand, if you relax, say by lying on a beach in the sun, you will find that your mind begins to drift vaguely around, not thinking of anything in particular, and the moment you do start thinking of something and focusing on it, you stop being relaxed. In contrast, when people are tense and anxious, they will usually complain that their minds run round and round and that they just cannot stop thinking about what is worrying them.

Hypnosis has the unusual characteristic of combining concentration with relaxation, which means that you can, for instance, focus on something which disturbs or distresses you and still be relaxed. This involves the process of splitting or separating different 'lines of consciousness'. Such an experience can break the link between an idea, memory or thought, and its attendant anxiety and tension. This, again, is an example of the *control* you have in hypnosis. In ordinary states of mind, the link between concentration and tension, physical or mental or both, is automatic; in hypnosis, you can separate the two, and learn how to do this in such a way as to become able to do it at will in everyday life.

I think it was Matthew Arnold who wrote in one of his books that a schoolboy, when asked to define faith, replied: 'Believing something that you know is not true'. Hypnosis can be something like that. Just as in the example described above (i.e. of feeling your arm becoming light), you can believe, for the time being, something that you actually know is impossible. For the time during which you believe whatever it is, for all practical purposes, it might as well *be* true. This actually happens a great deal in everyday life.

Take the example of a small child who has to go into hospital for an operation. Not very long ago, such a child would have been tucked into its hospital bed by its mother, who would then go away, and other people would come, total strangers to the child, who would do all sorts of strange, uncomfortable, even painful things to him. The child would not understand what on earth was going on. He would be frightened and confused, and would probably believe that Mummy had abandoned him, and that she did not care, did not love him, and would never come back. Probably the child would begin to think that he must have done something very bad to have made Mummy stop loving him. Children experiencing separation in the first few years of life come to believe just that, and can become severely depressed, either then or later in life. Even though most children appear to 'get over it', something deep inside them seems to go on believing that they are not loved, not secure, and that they are *bad* in some way that they cannot actually pin down, do not understand, and which, in consequence, is not under their control.

As far as such children, and the adults they grow into, are concerned, the belief that they are not loved, have been abandoned, and therefore are not lovable, can have exactly the same effects as if they actually *were* unloved. This can have grave and damaging effects later in life. In hypnosis, you may come to believe things which can have equally powerful effects.

To follow this example through, suppose that an adult who has had this sort of experience when a very small child, comes for help because he now has a strong feeling of being unlovable, worthless and so on. In hypnosis, he may be asked to believe that he is going backwards through time until he is, say, two years old again, and being taken to hospital. This technique is called 'age regression'. If he is good at hypnosis, he will regress to feeling two years old again, and again experience feeling helpless as his mother tucks him into this strange bed in a strange room and then goes away. He will feel all the emotions he felt when it actually happened, but this time, he is there observing in his adult mind as well, and so can understand what is going on in a way that he could not understand all those years ago. This is often enough to enable the person concerned to have a different perception of the experience and so 'let go' of it. You might say, then, the mere fact that, as an adult, he can remember the whole event in the normal way, should mean that he can understand it, but in fact, remembering and re-experiencing are not the same, and above all, do not *feel* the same. It is generally the feelings associated with very early experiences which we 'lose' or which get hidden away, not the memory of the event, although sometimes the memory of very painful events can become totally repressed.

If you re-experience an event like this, and therefore recover and go through all the feelings and thoughts that went with the original experience, you find that the memory changes, or rather, the influence it has, changes, and it changes because, for the time you were working on the experience, you *believed* that you were two years old, with all the feelings and ideas of that time, and yet at the same time you could apply your adult understanding.

To sum up, hypnosis is a natural experience that most people have had at some time. Almost all children use self-hypnosis in imaginative play, and almost all adults use their imagination, either deliberately or involuntarily, in just the way that hypnosis works. All that clinical hypnosis does is to mobilize a natural talent in practical and purposeful ways to improve physical and mental health. It is not magic, it has nothing to do with mysticism or the occult, and it is not related to any religion. In actual fact, all the major religions of the world have investigated hypnosis, because of the false ideas in the past about its moral and mystical character, and have approved it as a medical technique. Hypnosis does share some features with mystical and religious experiences, however, and is very like the state of deep meditation which is taught in some religious systems. Clinical hypnosis is nevertheless something different from all of these, and should never be thought of in any way other than as a thoroughly practical and down-to-earth technique that can be used for equally practical and down-to-earth treatment of all kinds of disorders, both physical and psychological.

Chapter 3

What Can Be Treated Through Hypnosis?

Hypnosis in itself, is not, as has been already emphasized, a treatment for anything. It is little more than a method of *administering* a treatment, a special way of carrying out a treatment which could be given without hypnosis. This means, of course, that the therapist using hypnosis must have a thorough knowledge of the condition or problem which he is attempting to treat, and of the principles and techniques of the treatment which he intends to apply through hypnosis. The skills and knowledge which are necessary if you are to be helped with either psychological or physical problems, or, or indeed both, are those of medicine, clinical psychology or some form of psychotherapy. A 'therapist' who uses hypnosis but who does not have appropriate training in one or more of these other disciplines is unlikely to be of any real help to anyone, and could in practice make things considerably worse.

However, when combined with the expertise of a trained person who has specialized in the area concerned, the right treatment approaches and methods with hypnosis can be very powerful. There is a psychological element in all physical illnesses and conditions. For instance, if you strain your back and find yourself in pain and unable to move freely, the pain actually protects you from further injury by limiting your movements and helps your recovery by allowing the muscles to relax and heal. At the same time, however, you will probably be somewhat alarmed by what has happend, and that alarm will tend to make you hold yourself stiffly and awkwardly. This in turn will tend to keep the muscles tense and so prolong the pain.

To take an even more serious example, most people undergoing surgery are frightened and anxious. Surgeons and nurses have known for a long time that these feelings delay recovery and prolong convalescence, and may even affect the degree of recovery. As a result, hospital staff nowadays take great care to prepare patients for operations by giving them information, by explaining the operation and its effects and by giving extensive reassurance. Understanding reduces anxiety and fear, and so reduces stress. Such practices have been proved to improve recovery, speed up rehabilitation, and reduce the amount of pain-killing drugs needed, as well as reducing distress and suffering.

Much the same is true of illness and injury of any kind. Fear, anxiety, physical and mental tension all militate against recovery, as well as making the perception of pain and discomfort more intense. Relaxation and the discharge of tension and fear can be especially well achieved by the use of hypnosis and hypnotic techniques.

It is well known that some conditions, such as asthma, eczema, psoriasis, migraine, and many others, are closely related to psychological stress and distress. In such conditions the relief of stress and anxiety can lead to a very welcome reduction in symptoms. Hypnotic techniques can assist such treatment and lead to very effective ways in which the sufferer is able to help him or herself to reduce the severity of the condition, and even sometimes to eliminate it. Similarly, psychological distress of any kind can often be more readily and more powerfully relieved using hypnosis than without. Grief can be put aside for a while, anxiety lessened, pre-occupying and worrying thoughts put on ice for a short period. Equally, more specialized treatments can be eased, or speeded up through various particular applications of hypnosis.

For example, many anxiety states or reactions that simply do not make sense in terms of the present-day life of the sufferer, stem from traumatic events much earlier in life, usually in childhood. Because those events or experiences were so very disturbing, they have been blocked from consciousness, and the person concerned simply cannot remember anything of that kind happening. As far as he is concerned, it never happened at all. He may be aware of the fact that something bad or frightening happened when he was, say, four years old, but has no idea at all what it might have been. Psychotherapy and psychoanalysis are used to treat such conditions with the aim of enabling the person to recover the memory of the event, and see it in perspective. This can take a long time, sometimes even several years of regular and frequent interviews. Using hypnosis, it is often possible to recover the memory and deal with it in just a few sessions, and do so with much less distress and disturbance.

Hypnosis on its own, or simply with suggestions of feeling good, relaxed and so on, is actually very pleasant. I thoroughly enjoy simply spending a little time in a trance from time to time, and so do those patients with whom I use hypnosis. After their first experience of entering the trance state, without any other work being done, they usually smile broadly as they return to the 'ordinary world', and say how good they feel. That experience can be very helpful if you are in pain, or anxious, or depressed, but it will make very little difference if any to what is really troubling you: that will have to be specifically dealt with in the course of further therapy.

Because hypnosis is so relaxing and comforting, it is of great help in treating anxiety and depression. In and of itself, it will not affect the underlying problems, but can make them easier to bear for a time. There is, however, more to it than just that. For instance, suppose you suffer from attacks of anxiety, which can occur anywhere and at any time. In those attacks, you may find that you feel terrified, or go into a panic; you feel your heart is racing; you feel hot and sweaty or cold and clammy; you may feel nauseated and become afraid you will faint. Once you have had a few attacks like this, perhaps in the street or in a shop, you then become frightened of an attack coming and so avoid going out. That apprehension, the fear that an attack may happen, in itself makes it more likely that you *will* get such an attack. The tension that the fear creates predisposes you to these reactions.

Spending some time in hypnosis every day will help you get rid of the build-up of tension and anxiety, and so make it much less likely that you will have such an attack. Still more helpful, though, is the way you can learn to use hypnosis to deal with an attack when it happens and stop it from disrupting your life. Finally, hypnosis may make it much easier and quicker to discover what the cause or causes of the problem may be, such as a forgotten or 'repressed' traumatic memory, as described above, and so help you free yourself of it, so that you no longer have the attacks at all.

Many different emotional and psychological difficulties and problems can be treated using hypnosis to speed treatment up and make it easier to cope with. Hypnosis can be a great help in treating some sexual problems, obsessional habits, temper outbursts, and so on. Not all conditions can be treated in such ways; some depressed states, for instance, are better treated in other ways.

One of the earliest uses of hypnosis was to lessen or even eliminate pain. In the days before anaesthetics, any surgery was an ordeal, sometimes absolutely agonizing. As in the story of Jacob Grimm told in Chapter 1, anything that holds the attention of the patient really firmly can help to reduce or even suppress all awareness of pain. Dr Esdaile used hypnotic anaesthesia on hundreds of patients undergoing surgery when he worked in India in the nineteenth century. The accounts of his experiences, when he published them, were not believed by his colleagues back in Europe. Nowadays, many dentists use hypnosis both to help their patients feel calm and relaxed and to ensure that they feel no pain from the dental work. Hypnotic anaesthesia and analgesia (reduction of pain) are being used increasingly throughout the world in all kinds of surgical procedures, from the smallest stitching to really major operations.

In Britain, it is still unusual for surgeons to use hypno-anaesthesia, but hypnotic techniques have been used for a very long time by midwives and obstetricians, although they do not usually call such methods by that name. The relaxation exercises that mothers-to-be are commonly taught in ante-natal classes produce, in those women that can manage it, a state of light hypnosis, which enables them to cope with labour much more easily and with less pain than otherwise.

Another growing application of hypnotic techniques is with children who have been injured in accidents, especially if they have suffered burns, both in order to make the necessary treatments less painful and to reduce the effect of the injury. While hypno-anaesthesia is still not very commonly used in Britain, more and more people are being trained in its use, and the practice is spreading.

A report written by Dr Abney M. Ewin of the Medical School at Tulane University, USA, gives a good illustration of how hypnosis can work. In a privately circulated report, he describes how he works in the Medical School Hospital. When a patient is brought into Emergency with extensive and severe burns, he, or one of the other doctor's trained in hypnosis, is called immediately. While emergency dressings are being applied and drips put up, the hypnotherapist introduces himself, and, after obtaining the patient's agreement to the use of hypnosis, asks him to describe a favourite place, which he then calls the 'laughing place'. The therapist then carries out a very quick induction of hypnosis, and tells the patient to go to his 'laughing place', so distracting the patient from awareness of both pain and fear. Finally, he talks to the patient about the burned part of his body beginning to feel cool and comfortable, and the pain and burning feelings becoming less and less. The patient is encouraged to stay in hypnosis, and therefore in his 'laughing place', until all the painful and distressing emergency treatments have been finished. The patient is also taught how to enter hypnosis on his own so that he can go to his 'laughing place' whenever dressings are replaced or other painful procedures carried out. Patients treated in this way feel much less pain and are less frightened and disturbed by the experiences they have to undergo in hospital. Even more impressive is the fact that the burns do not develop in the usual way or produce the normal severe physical and physiological reactions, require much less treatment and heal more quickly and completely.

Another condition that hypnosis can very effectively help with is high blood-pressure. Some specialists now encourage patients to learn how to control their own blood-pressure by 'Bio-Feedback Training'. This is done by measuring the patient's blood-pressure at short intervals, using a device that shows the patient very plainly in figures what is happening from minute to minute. Then the patient is trained to relax in one way or another, and he will see that, as he becomes relaxed, his blood-pressure drops. Similarly, when he lets himself become excited, or thinks about something that has been worrying him, he will see his blood-pressure rise again. This makes it very clear to the patient that what he thinks and feels, and how he generally manages his life, has a major bearing on what happens in his arteries. Even more helpful is the fact that, with some experience using a machine like this, the patient begins to learn how he *feels* when his blood-pressure goes up and when it goes down, so that he can begin to gain control over it in every day life without the machine.

The same approach is used with hypnotherapy for hypertension, but generally the effect is quicker and easier for those patients who take well to hypnosis. Additionally, spending two or three periods of ten minutes or so in the deeply relaxed state of the hypnotic trance has in itself a beneficial effect on high blood-pressure. Many heart conditions too can be helped in this way, the reduction of the accumulated tensions that we all have helping to reduce the effects of the heart defect and so making the patient's life safer and more comfortable, and at the same time reducing the stresses on the heart itself.

Stomach disorders, intestinal problems and any malfunction of the digestive tract can be helped through hypnosis. Sometimes, just as in the case of high blood-pressure and some heart problems, it is chronic and accumulating tension that is the root of the problem, and hypnotic relaxation can reduce this build-up with good effects on the organs affected. It can be helpful to use hypnosis to explore unconscious feelings and memories that underlie the anxiety, in addition to the relaxation and easing of tension.

Every organ in the body is affected by one's emotions and experiences, and in turn, the way we feel, and the way we experience our lives and react to the events in them, is affected by what is happening physically in our organs. All forms of counselling and psychotherapy can be helpful even in the most obviously physical disorders, which is why physicians, surgeons and nurses nowadays spend much more time talking with their patients than was usual in the days before we began to recognize the intimate interaction of the physical, mental and emotional aspects of our lives. For the same reason, hypnosis can be a very effective way of intervening in the vicious cycle of anxiety – physical or chemical malfunction – pain – more anxiety, which is a major factor in the origin, development and maintenance of all kinds of physical illness.

Then there are all sorts of other, less dramatic but often just as important, areas in which we might need help. Hypnosis can be used very effectively to help you give up smoking, to make it easier to stick to a diet, to deal with compulsive eating, to stop biting your nails, and many other habitual actions. Hypnosis can also be used very effectively for improving your concentration and attention. For example, when preparing for an examination, the anxiety of the impending ordeal may actually make it more difficult to study effectively and to remember what you are revising. If each session of revision is started by ten minutes in hypnosis, letting your mind become clear and relaxed, and reminding yourself that you are perfectly capable of absorbing the knowledge you need, that you have actually learned it all before and all you are doing is refreshing your memory, then you will reap considerably greater benefit from your study time than if you approached it anxiously and tensely. Many students can testify also to the boon of being able to 'cure' their own exam nerves. One of the first students to ask for my help in this way, is a good example. In fact, it was not she but her mother who asked me for help! The young lady in question had made life hell for the whole family for about three weeks before every major examination. She was coming up to a particularly important examination, and her mother could not bear the thought of what the next few weeks would be like. The girl was a very good hypnotic subject and learnt to take herself into a trance very quickly. During the weeks before the examinations, she practised it regularly, using imagery specifically designed to reduce her anxiety reaction to the thought of exams, the room in which the exams were to be held, and so on. When the due date came, she became very unpopular with her friends because she was so relaxed, and, perhaps, unsympathetic about their anxiety!

Always, however, one must remember that hypnosis is not the treatment itself. It is merely the means through which the treatment is given. After all, when you are treated by a doctor for an infection and he gives you an injection, it is what is *inside* the syringe that cures the infection. If there were nothing in the syringe, or just sterilized water, the only benefit you would receive is what is called the 'placebo effect'. You might feel better, and perhaps even recover more quickly than if you had not had the injection, but the infection itself would not be affected by the sterile water. Hypnosis is like the needle and syringe: it does not treat your problem, merely conveys the treatment to you. Hypnosis is often a quicker and more effective way of administering the treatment, just as a hypodermic injection may be a quicker and more effective way of getting the drug to work than a tablet taken by mouth. But, just as with a hypodermic syringe, there is a placebo effect: it makes you feel better because you feel something is being done about your problem.

There is actually something of a paradox about all this. Being given an injection of something without any medical power or chemical or physiological effect, or taking a pill composed entirely of a neutral substance, *does* make you feel better. Furthermore, given such a non-treatment, you will probably recover more quickly than if you had been given nothing at all. This effect makes medical research notoriously difficult. Whenever a new drug is developed and tested, it has to be compared with a neutral substance as well as with existing drugs. If the patients who are being treated with a new drug *know* that it is new, they will show considerably greater response to it than to their old medication. So they have to be given a 'placebo' (Latin for 'I shall please'), which also is presented as the new drug for comparison.

It seems that, even with the most sophisticated and powerful drugs, faith, or belief in the efficacy of the drug, is very important. The same thing is true of hypnosis. If you believe that hypnosis is going to make you feel better, then that belief will enhance the pleasant feelings you will experience while you are in the trance and that linger on afterwards.

This 'placebo effect' really seems to be a treatment in itself. It is not just that you feel better after the neutral pill, injection or whatever, or after the short hypnotic trance you have experienced: you do get better more quickly than if you had had no treatment at all. Somehow, the ritual of receiving a treatment in which you believe, and from which you expect good things, seems to mobilize your inner resources and speed up the natural healing of whatever is amiss.

Doctors will never use a placebo, that is, a totally neutral substance, pretending it is a drug, in clinical practice, if the patient they are treating genuinely needs specific treatment. Similarly, when using hypnosis, a doctor or psychologist will never present the induction of a trance as a treatment. The fact that spending time in hypnosis is pleasant, and that it facilitates recovery from whatever is troubling you, is not enough to qualify it as treatment. Its generally beneficial effects are a bonus. Unlike many medicines, it does not have to taste awful if it is to do you any good! But it is the work that is done *during* the hypnotic state which is the treatment.

Chapter 4

How Does Hypnosis Work?

Philosophers throughout recorded history have struggled to understand the way that mind and body co-exist. Many people have found it difficult to understand the relationship between these two aspects of what it is to be human. Those who believe in spirit or soul have struggled with the added complication this brings to the problem of the relationships between these three: body, mind, spirit. From time to time, individual thinkers have tried to cut through these problems by proposing that mind and body are a single, united, and mortal, whole, while the human spirit is believed to be immortal. This concept, that there is no separation between the two aspects (mind and body) of humanness, has become more and more accepted over the last few decades. The term 'holistic medicine' has been created to describe theories and practices of health and illness that regard what happens in bodily processes and what happens in the mind as being all of a piece.

It has been well known for a long time that bodily processes, whether chemical, electrical or mechanical, affect mental processes and state. For instance, it is difficult to concentrate properly when the concentration of sugars in your blood-stream falls below its usual level, as, for example, when a long time has passed since you have eaten and you feel very hungry. Probably, too, your mood will change, either for the better or for the worse, when you allow alcohol to enter your blood-stream. As the concentration of alcohol in the blood rises your mood changes more and more, your thinking becomes less precise and sensible, and you may lose control of your limbs, until eventually you lose consciousness altogether. Or, again, if you experience a massive blow to the head, you will lose consciousness, and if it was really severe, you may find, when you come round again, that you cannot remember what happened for some period of time before the blow. The effects that physical processes and experiences can have on mental and emotional experiences are utilized in psychiatry. For example, passing an electric current through the brain is a treatment sometimes used to treat really severe depressive illnesses, and can be very effective indeed. Many valuable drugs used in psychiatry change our mental processes, modifying such experiences as hallucinations and delusions, or moods such as chronic anxiety or depression by affecting the way that nerves conduct electrical currents in the brain.

This process clearly works the other way round. As we have noted already, the thoughts and feelings you have in your mind will affect the way your body functions. For example, if you become tense, anxious or perhaps frightened, one of the first things that happens is that your body reacts by releasing adrenaline into the blood stream. The effects of this hormone combine to make the body more ready to act vigorously either by fighting or running away. One of the ways it does this is by reducing the blood-flow to the stomach and intestines, and increasing it to the muscles to help you either to fight or run more efficiently and powerfully, and in extreme cases makes you empty your bladder and bowels. It also causes your heart to pump blood more strongly around your body, your breathing to become faster, and sweat to break out, especially on the palms of your hands. By contrast, when you are content, your muscles relax, your heart-rate is slow and steady, and you breathe freely and easily.

Increasingly, both in the fields of medicine and psychology on the one hand, and in theology, philosophy and related fields on the other, people are abandoning the concept of dualism (that is, that mind and body are separate although interacting) and are coming to think of a human being as a united, integrated or single *whole* – hence the term 'holistic'.

Hypnotherapy employs an understanding of Man which is founded on the idea that anything that happens in the mind also happens in the body, and that anything that happens in the body also happens in the mind. Every thought or feeling you experience is manifested or shown in some bodily change or action. Similarly, every process in your body, or anything that happens to it, will necessarily have mental aspects, that is, perceptions, thoughts, and feelings associated with it.

When working in this way, therefore, we believe that in using mental processes to produce change in the mind, we are necessarily creating changes in the body also. The same, of course, is true the other way round: if we approach a patient with physical treatments, mental changes will necessarily occur.

There are many different concepts of holistic medicine or therapy. Some of them are little more than disguised forms of the old dualism, or sometimes 'triolism'. For instance, I know an orthopaedic surgeon, a very devout and sincere Christian, who believes, as I do, that a broken leg is not just a physical event in the body, but an event in the whole person. When he sees a patient with a broken leg, he therefore does not just re-set the bone, plaster the leg and prescribe painkillers and antibiotics. He also spends time talking with the patient, trying to explain what has happened physically, what the treatment will do, and reassuring and advising on all aspects of the situation. He also will pray with the patient and the other staff assisting in the treatment. In doing all this, he is trying to involve every aspect of the patient as a person, his whole being, in the treatment and in the healing process.

This is not holistic treatment, although it is a lot nearer to it than the way many doctors used to work. My friend's approach recognizes that a human being is not just a body that you can mend like a broken chair, but that the physical accident involves more than the bone, and more even than simply the rest of the body. My friend, however, thinks of his patient as a spiritual being which exists within a physical body through the mediation of a mind. This is not a single *whole*, but a trinity, within which the body and mind are only vehicles for the spirit. Holistic thinking regards the patient as an organic or living *single* organism in which nothing is separate or divided, and in which physical events, such as pain, digestion, breathing, sleeping, etc. themselves, are only *aspects* of the events that are taking place. Similarly, mental processes, remembering, learning, repeating the times tables, feeling sad, feeling happy, or angry or frightened, loving, hating etc., are only *aspects* of the whole event that is taking place.

Think, for example, of a piece of wood, three inches thick, three inches wide and six inches long. It is painted matt white. Imagine it on top of a pedestal, so that it is at the same height as your eyes. Shine a clear white light on it. Look at it from one end, and you will see a white square, three inches each way. Now stand it up on end and look at it again: you will see a white rectangle, six inches by three. Now change the lighting to a pure red and bring someone else into the room, and ask them what they see. They will tell you they see a red rectangle, six inches by three, or a red square, three inches by three, depending on the angle from which they are looking.

What *is* there on the pedestal? A square, a rectangle, a block? Is it white, or red, or what? What you see and how you think of it depends on your line of vision, on the light you are seeing by, and your distance from the block. Yet in the end, what you actually *have*, is a block of matt white wood, six inches by three inches by three inches.

That is how the holistic therapist tries to think about people, not perhaps as blocks of wood, but as complete wholes of which we can see only certain aspects at any one time, depending on our viewpoint and the level of our understanding. And that, ideally, is the framework of thinking in which we use hypnosis and in which it works best.

In practice what the therapist will do is to show you how to make changes in one aspect of what is going, or has gone, wrong. The effect of this will be to change the way that the whole *system*, which is you, functions, and to do it in such a way as to reduce or remove the problem which is troubling you, or to change the effect the problem has on your life.

We can now look at various hypnotic techniques in more details. Symptoms, pain, and other problems, can be approached in a variety of ways in hypnosis, using one or more of the different characteristics of the hypnotic state. In an earlier chapter, a spontaneous form of hypnosis was described as it occurs in the lives of many people: the experience of driving a car while one is unaware for a period of time of even *being in* the car. In normal circumstances, we can think of several things at the same time, and be aware of all of them simultaneously. We are, at those times, following several lines of consciousness all at once, and can switch attention from one line to another as needed. For example, while knitting, watching television and chatting all at the same time, you may come to a more difficult part of your knitting pattern. You may then ask the people with whom you are talking to be quiet for a moment, you avert your eyes from the TV and mentally close your ears to the sound, while you pay close attention to the problem with your knitting. Once the problem is solved, you can take up the conversation again and pay further attention to the TV programme.

When you enter an hypnotic state, however, either spontaneously perhaps without even noticing, or in response to an induction that a therapist is presenting, then the various lines of consciousness, which have been.discussed in Chapter 2, can begin to separate and lose contact with each other. Your attention, and your whole awareness, will gradually narrow down until it is focussed along one channel only. At the same time, although you may not be conscious of it, you will probably keep up a separate channel of attention to all the other things of which you are normally conscious. That is to say, the sounds from outside the room, the tightness of your shoes, the shopping or other work you have to do later in the day, will all be monitored, but in your central consciousness, you will not think about or notice any of these sensations and thoughts.

Suppose that you have a chronic pain, where either the cause is more or less permanent and cannot be treated, or where the treatment to reduce the cause of the pain will take a long time.

This might, for example, be something like degeneration of a spinal disc, or arthritic changes in your joints. You have probably been taking painkillers, and may not want to continue having to use them. In hypnosis, you will still feel the pain. Simply suggesting that the pain disappears would probably have no effect, or if it did, this will not work for more than a short time. It *is* possible, however, to assign the pain to a line of consciousness that is separate from your central awareness, so that, just as, in our example above, you are not aware of driving or of all the sensations and perceptions involved in that complex set of actions, you may become unaware of the pain, and cease to notice it. As far as you are concerned, therefore, the pain has gone. The pain is still there, but you simply do not notice it.

This happens naturally in various situations. For example, it has frequently been reported that soldiers, in the middle of a fierce bout of fighting can receive severe injuries and can be completely oblivious of the fact that they have been hurt, until either the fighting dies away and they can rest for a moment, or someone else points out to them that they are injured, whereupon they feel the pain as fully as they would under normal circumstances. The same thing sometimes happens in the excitement of a game of football, when a player may not realize that he has been hurt until the game is over, when he notices the injury and the pain associated with it. He may have no idea of when or how he was injured. Throughout the battle or the game, attention is so exclusively focused on the activity involved and the intense arousal generated by the situation, that the pain messages simply do not enter conciousness. In hypnosis, therefore, we can assign the pain to a different, and less immediate, level of awareness.

The technique of occupying the attention of the individual so strongly and exclusively on a chosen topic so that all other aspects of the present are ignored, was illustrated by the story of Jacob Grimm's childhood operation. Hypnosis can be used in the same way. It is rather terrifying to think of lying on the operating table while the surgical team operates on your body while you are awake and aware of what is going on. Yet many minor and major operations can be, and are, carried out with no anaesthesia other than hypnosis.

How does this work? How can you be lying on the operating table having very painful things done to you without feeling any pain and without being at least a little alarmed as to what is going on? Imagine the following situation.

You have been booked to have an operation. Before that date, you meet the hypnotherapist (who might be the surgeon himself, the anaesthetist, a nurse, or a psychologist) who teaches you how to go into the hypnotic state and practises with you on perhaps several occasions. He teaches you also that when he says, 'Now go to your private place', you will find yourself in a place that you have discussed with him, a place you remember with the happiest and most relaxed feelings. It might be a scene from childhood, or from a holiday, your wedding day, anything. You learn how to become so absorbed in that picture that you simply do not notice anything else. When you come into the operating theatre at last, you know what to do, and when the hypnotherapist leads you into hypnosis and then says, 'Now go to your private place', you go there in your mind and simply do not see the theatre or the surgeon and nurses any more. And similarly you do not feel what is being done to your body because you are on a beach, or snuggled up to your mother while she sings you a lullaby, or whatever else you have chosen.

Another approach, both to pain and to other problems, is to use imagery by means of which body functions may be altered, This, too, is based on events that happen in everyday life. When I was in my early teens, I used to go touring on a bicycle, and camp overnight. One evening I asked at a farm if I might pitch my tent in the corner of a field. The farmer insisted there was no need to use the tent, and that I should sleep in the unused milking-parlour just behind the farmhouse. When night came, I bedded down in a corner of this building, close to the door, the upper half of which I left open. During the night I happened to wake, and looking out through the open half-door, I saw the silhouette of a monk, apparently looking in at me. I was terrified. Until that moment, I had not believed in ghosts, but I became an instant believer! I lay, petrified, unable to move a single muscle, my heart beating more than twice its normal rate, with sweat breaking out over my whole body. After some time, which seemed like hours, I gradually noticed that the silhouette was absolutely stationary. Then it dawned on me that what I was looking at was the silhouette of the shed next to the milking-parlour, and not a ghostly monk at all. My heart slowed down, the sweat dried, and I could move again!

What you hold in your mind and what you believe, affects all aspects of your being. If you believe something frightening is present, you become afraid, with all the physical responses of that reaction. If you believe you have won the pools, you will become happy and excited, with, again, all the responses typical of that state. Suppose then, that with all the intensification of attention, concentration and absorption that hypnosis provides, you picture yourself lowering one hand into a container of ice-cold water. You picture the lumps of ice floating on the water, and that you are pushing them aside with your hand as you put it in the water, feelings its icy touch. You feel the cold seeping into your hand, gradually numbing it until your hand feels totally numb, with no sensation other than cold. If, at that point, someone else were to touch your hand, you probably would not feel the touch. You probably would not even feel a needle pricking your hand. Your hand would, as far as you were concerned, be totally numb.

Then you put that numb hand over whatever part of your body is in pain, and feel the numbness seeping from your hand into the other body part, until that too is cold and numb. As the painful part of your body gradually goes cold and numb, the pain fades away.

The picture of the icy water, and your hand immersed in it, becoming cold itself, is simply a way of incorporating the idea that your hand is going numb, so that your whole mind will accept the process. Some people can manage to achieve this effect without the picture, but you need to have an unusually good 'hypnotic talent' to do it like that, and most of us need the help of a mental image. Once you have accepted the idea, then the rest follows: your hand loses all sensation, just as it would if cooled in this way.

Not only are actual sensations modified by images such as this while they are held in the mind, but other bodily functions can be altered in the same way. For instance, a severe burn will not produce blisters, inflammation, or any of the normal physiological responses to burning, if you hold in your mind a clear and vivid image of the burned parts being cool and comfortable. The use of this, in Emergency Departments, as described by Dr Ewin, has already been mentioned in Chapter 3.

Similar techniques can be used for reducing high blood-pressure. An image or picture is built up of the blood-vessels in your body, perhaps as hoses, with the blood flowing through them with difficulty because the hoses are stiff and tight. This image is then gradually modified by imagining that the hoses are softening, so that the blood can travel down them more easily and smoothly. In addition, suggestions will be made that the pressure inside is being relieved by the hoses becoming soft and stretchy. As this changing image is developed, so your actual blood-pressure really does drop. What you hold in your mind is a part of your whole being and so is reflected in and affects all other aspects of your being.

Skin conditions such as eczema or psoriasis can sometimes also be improved with images. For instance, some cases of eczema are improved by sunshine. To the surprise of the sufferer, 'imaginary' sunshine in hypnosis is just as effective as the real thing!

One patient of mine can provide a very vivid illustration of this technique. At not quite five years of age, Linda (not her real name) had suffered from really severe eczema since her second week of life. It was so bad that she had had to have continuous treatment with cortico-steroids from the time she was two weeks old, with the attendant danger that she would not grow or mature properly. Despite this treatment, the itching she experienced was so intense she had to be given sedatives every day of her life. Even so, no one in the family had had a whole night's sleep since she was born, because she scratched herself so deeply at night that she would wake in intense pain, lying, as her parents put it, in a pool of blood. Finally, because of the scratching, she had be on continuous treatment by antibiotics to avoid infections. Her parents told me that moderately cool water seemed to be only thing that stopped the otherwise continuous and intense irritation, but that when Linda got into a bath, the deep scratches and splits in her skin would sting so much it was almost worse than the itching itself.

Linda told me, when we first met and talked generally, that she liked fairies and cats, and agreed with me that she would love to go to Fairy Land. I told her that I knew a way in which she could go to Fairy Land if she did what I would teach her. There she would meet a special Fairy who would help her make her skin stop itching and help it to heal. Linda decided this was a good idea. I began an induction of hypnosis, and soon she felt herself floating away carried under a balloon which was taking her to Fairy Land. When she arrived there, she was met by her special Fairy and a cat.

The Fairy took her hand and led her to a beautiful patch of grass, surrounded by trees and flowers. In the middle of the grass area was a pool of magic water. I told Linda to kneel down and put one hand in the water, and that she should notice how the water was just pleasantly cool, just right to soothe the itching away. She could smooth the water onto any part of her that was itching, and the itching would stop.

I let her enjoy this scene for a little while. It was quite obvious, from the happy smiles which came from time to time, that she was indeed enjoying the experience! Then I asked her to leave Fairy Land, come back to my room and open her eyes. When she did so, she began to giggle, and then explained that the water had been so nice that she had decided to plunge right into it and splash about! She was quite definite in her assertion that the water stopped the itching completely. I then taught her how to take herself into the hypnotic state so that she could go to Fairy Land for a little while every day, and use the magic water to stop the itching, and at the same time, to help her skin heal.

Linda came to see me again a week later. She had practised her self-hypnosis every day, especially at bed time, and it had worked. Her parents told me that they had stopped all the medication, and that Linda no longer scratched at all. Whenever she felt an itch, she did something else I had taught her: simply to put one hand over the itching part, and think about the magic water. In this way, she was able to free herself completely of the distressing itch, and so avoid the scratching which had further damaged her skin in the past. I saw Linda very occasionally over the following year, and then largely because she was so keen to tell her 'magic doctor' the latest ideas she had had, and how her skin was getting better. By the end of the year her skin was astonishingly better, and she had even begun to produce sweat. This in itself represented a major step forward in the healing process, and augured well for the future.

There have been reports also of cancers responding more rapidly and completely to radiotherapy if that treatment is accompanied by imagery. For instance, the radiation is visualized as bullets hitting the growth and breaking off and killing the cancerous cells; the dead cells are then swallowed up and destroyed by the white cells in the blood-stream.

In more obviously psychological conditions the same effects can be found. Anxiety states, for instance, can be reduced in many sufferers by imagery, induced under hypnosis, of places and times in which there was nothing but calm, relaxation and peace. All anxiety problems can be reduced in susceptible patients, either by simple hypnotic relaxation or imagery. Some forms of depression can be lightened, again by visualizing some happy and relaxed experience, real or imaginary, or by visualizing the depressed feelings in some tangible form and then getting rid of the image which represents the feelings. For instance, I sometimes ask my patients to picture their feelings of unhappiness, hopelessness and despair as a dark, heavy oily liquid that fills them and weighs them down, making all thought, reaction and movement difficult and sluggish. They should then picture this heavy liquid gradually leaking away, draining out of their body like water leaking out of the holes in a bucket, and as it leaks away, so they feel themselves becoming lighter and lighter. Alternatively, I may suggest that they picture their worries, fears and miseries all written down on bits of paper. One by one, they take out the bits of paper, read what is written on each one, screw it up and then throw it into a river or into a fire so that each worry or misery is destroyed.

Many of the problems for which people seek help stem from things that happened to them earlier in life. Sometimes these events can be remembered, but thinking about them only seems to make things worse. More often the events concerned have been completely forgotten, or the feelings belonging to the events seem to have been blocked out. Hypnosis can be used to uncover such hidden memories or feelings. Remember, whatever you believe may as well be true, because it has the same effects as though it were true. This means that past experiences which were misunderstood because you were very young at the time, or were misperceived (like my hooded monk!), can be damaging to you, even if the actual event was quite harmless. Simply trying to remember the event, and thinking about it, if you can recall it, is unlikely to make much difference. However, if you re-experience the episode under hypnosis, and picture it as happening here and now, then your adult understanding really comes to bear on the memory trace, and you may find yourself freed from the effects that it had on you subsequent life.

Imagine for instance, that in an hypnotic trance you accept the idea that you are going backwards through time in order to re-experience something that happened to you many years ago. You may not even know what the event was, but you are going to go back to the very first time in your life that you experienced certain feelings. You will, if you are susceptible to hypnosis, and want this to happen, be able to let yourself go back in time: back through your own life, to the moment when indeed you first experienced these feelings. You may find this moment is one of which you were, until now, totally unaware; that is, it had been lost to memory. In this procedure, however, you will be able to experience it as vividly as though it were actually happening now. The event concerned might be in your childhood or even when you were a tiny baby, but it will certainly be an event that impressed itself very deeply on you. Sometimes the event was not perhaps actually a bad one, but seemed so to your childhood self, and so affected you accordingly.

For example, a young man came to me because he felt so desperately unhappy and a failure, despite the fact that everything in his life seemed to be highly successful and pleasant. He had been adopted as a tiny baby, and was, so he believed, completely happy about his adoption and loved his adopted parents. We started looking for early experiences in which he had had the despairing feelings that made his life such a misery. Without either of us expecting anything in particular, he found himself re-experiencing an event at which he had been a toddler, when a woman he and his mother met in the street had reacted quite strongly to hearing he was adopted. He burst into tears at this point, and when we discussed the experience he had just been through, he expressed the feeling that he must have buried all sorts of unhappy feelings about his adoption for all the years since then. This discovery seemed to be the turning point in his treatment: quite soon after that he felt so much more confident and hopeful that he felt able to end treatment.

On the other hand, the event to which you go back may have been really traumatic, even intolerably distressing, and so was blocked from normal memory. The deeply buried memory of that event, even though wholly unconscious, can affect your development, your thinking and feeling, and all your responses to the world in which you live. For example, a woman who had been sexually assaulted when about six years old by her father, told me that she could remember this event quite clearly. Naturally, the memory troubled her intensely, but she felt that there was something else that was worse.

Under hypnosis she went back to the first time she had been molested. She described the experience, with great distress, and then went on to tell me that she ran to her mother and told her.

Her mother, however, instead of doing something to comfort and protect the child, told her that she was being naughty, that she had a filthy mind, and that 'Daddies don't do things like that'. Mother sent the child off to her bedroom as a punishment. That seemed to be even more hurtful and destructive to my patient than the acts of her father had been. It took a very long time for her to work through all the feelings this recovered memory exposed.

Sometimes simply recovering such a memory and its associated feelings can unlock your problem. More usually, more work has to be done in order to take the damaging power out of the memory, and enable you to resolve the problems it created for you. Hypno-analysis, as this approach to such problems is called, may take many sessions, some with hypnosis and some without, to work through all that emerges from the locked-away recesses of memory. Sometimes the memories are so unacceptable and distressing that it might take several sessions to uncover them a little at a time. The process may have to be a slow one so that your consciousness can accept the memories without such distress as to make the whole experience hurt you even more. In fact, we usually find that if a memory recovered in hypnosis in this way is too distressing the patient simply does not remember it at the end of the session. Only when the whole mind is ready to receive the memory again, does it actually return completely.

Very occasionally a problem, whether manifested in a physical symptom or a psychological difficulty, responds to just a few sessions of treatment in hypnosis, and the patient is free of it again. More often, even if only a few sessions are needed with the therapist, you will have to continue working at the problem yourself, sometimes for a very long time. For instance, if you have high blood-pressure which you have learned to control through hypnosis, you will have to go on with regular and frequent sessions of self-hypnosis to keep it under control. I have already repeatedly insisted that hypnosis is not itself a treatment but simply a means of *giving* treatment. The next point is that treatment in hypnosis is rarely a cure, but rather a means of making adjustments in your whole being, which, like the adjustments made to a car when it is serviced, have to be repeated regularly in order to *keep* things working properly.

Patients are often disappointed that they are not cured by the treatment they receive, or disappointed when the treatment goes on working only if they keep up their sessions of self-hypnosis. In fact, there is more they still have to do: and that is, to change those aspects of their life styles that not only created the problem but have maintained it. Hypnosis may deal very effectively with the acute symptoms and provide techniques for dealing with some of the causes, if these are understood. Sometimes it can even provide the means of resolving the cause of a problem, especially if this lies in unconscious memory. More often than not, however, the symptoms from which we suffer are created and certainly maintained by a whole host of additional factors. These will involve our relationships with our families and friends (*and* our enemies); the ways in which we bottle up our feelings and the ways in which we express them; our work; the ways in which we spend our leisure time; the ways in which we sit, stand, and breathe; our diet; the exercise we take (or more often, do not take); and the place where we live. In other words, it is the whole pattern of the day-to-day ways in which we lead our lives that helps to determine the difficulties and problems for which we may seek help and treatment. Until and unless we identify and then change the things that contribute so intimately to our disease, we are not really taking responsibility for our own health. Unless we deal with those things that put us under stress, any 'cure' will be only temporary.

Sometimes a major aspect of what is wrong is unchangeable, such as, for instance, arthritic changes in joints, a collapsed spinal disc, an amputated limb, an unalterable but unsatisfactory relationship, or whatever; then a cure is impossible. You will have to go on working at controlling the symptoms, whether they be physical discomfort or mental pain, for a very long time. Hypnosis will help if you use it and go on using it regularly, but it will not provide a magical solution.

Chapter 5

What Is It Like?

What is it like to be hypnotized? The fact that we commonly experience spontaneous hypnotic states in everyday life in a variety of ways, has already been mentioned several times. However, what you experience in a session of formal hypnosis will seem very similar in some ways and very different in others. Patients sometimes remark after their first session on the fact that what happened, and what they felt, was very like something that they have experienced before of their own accord and without thinking of it as hypnosis. Others will say that it was quite different from what they expected and completely new to them.

Hypnosis is not the same as sleep, and has little if anything to do with it, except that dreams and hypnosis have a lot in common. However, going into an hypnotic trance is actually very like drifting into sleep. Going into hypnosis is therefore very familiar, as we all know what going to sleep is like. Being in a trance is, as you will now realize, also very familiar, and yet most people after their first experience of formal hypnosis feel surprised because they had not expected it to be 'like that'.

Perhaps the best way of giving you a picture of what you might expect if you were to ask for hypnosis, would be to describe a fairly typical interview with a doctor or psychologist who is going to help you to use hypnosis to deal with some problem that has been troubling you. Naturally it is impossible to describe how *your* therapist will work. Every therapist has his own approach, and no two will use the same methods, images, and procedures, but the following will be fairly typical.

The first step is likely to be a discussion of what you and your therapist are going to try and do, and how you are going to approach it. You may be asked what you know about hypnosis. If you have any misconceptions, they should be corrected. The therapist will probably tell you much the same sort of things about hypnosis as you have been reading in this book. He will explain how you will be conscious the whole time, that you will remember all you want to, and that you will be able to speak or move or do anything else you may want to do while you are in hypnosis.

You may then be asked about your happiest experiences, and to identify one special time and place when you really felt that 'all's right with the world', a moment and place in your life when everything was trouble-free and you felt completely happy and relaxed. You will probably be asked also if there are any situations or images that you especially dislike or that might disturb you. For instance, if you have hay-fever, and then were to be asked in hypnosis to imagine yourself in a country meadow in summer, you would probably find yourself beginning to sneeze. Or perhaps you may have a fear of lifts, and therefore would not be at all comfortable at being asked to picture yourself stepping into a lift. The therapist will usually try to ensure that he does not use any images which might cause you distress or make it difficult for you to continue with the session.

When this preliminary discussion is complete, you may be asked to fix your eyes on a spot on the ceiling or on the wall and stare at it as hard as you can. While you do that, the therapist will suggest that you begin to relax. He may ask you to notice what sensations you feel, and to let yourself drift away, rather as though you were drifting into sleep, but still remaining alert and listening to what he says. You will probably find at this stage that your eyes begin to get tired and strained, and you will find yourself blinking. The therapist may mention this, and add that after a little while you will find your eyes closing as though by themselves. He may suggest that when your eyes close in this way you will feel yourself relaxing even more and beginning to leave the everyday world behind you. This process of guiding you into 'disconnecting' from the here and now is called an induction.

As this progresses, you will feel more and more comfortable physically, and probably also feel increasingly peaceful and detached from the ordinary world. You might very well notice that any sounds from outside the room seem to be coming from further away, and they might even seem to fade away altogether. You will probably feel yourself becoming comfortably warm, even if it is a cold day, and you may notice your breathing becoming even, deep and regular. All this feels very like dropping gently off to sleep, and yet at the same time you will feel wide awake, and the therapist's voice will be completely clear to you. You will find yourself occasionally thinking of other things, but if you try, you will be able to ignore these distractions and become as absorbed in what the therapist is saying as you would be in an exciting or moving book or film.

You may, however, find yourself quite suddenly becoming anxious for a moment or two, and feeling very much in two minds about going ahead with the whole business. Very often we anticipate that anything new and unknown, like one's first experience of hypnosis, is likely to be a little alarming and even unnerving. If you feel like this you might find yourself opening your eyes, and saying something like: 'I don't think this is going to work'. Alternatively, you may feel you must not let the therapist down, and so you may restrain yourself from saying anything, even if you do feel disturbed. The best thing to do if you do feel anxious or uneasy, is to tell the therapist just what you are experiencing, so that he can help you deal with it.

There are different levels of hypnosis, just as there are different degrees of abstraction, concentration, or relaxation, and similar different depths of sleep. As you begin to go into trance, your hypnotic state will begin by being 'shallow' or 'light', but it can become 'deeper' or 'more profound'. Most authorities consider that there are three main grades or levels of trance: shallow, moderate, and deep. In actual fact, these levels are not really distinct or separated in any way; they grade one into the next imperceptibly. In a shallow trance, you can rouse yourself instantly simply by choosing to do so. In a moderately deep trance it would take you a moment or two to organize yourself into arousal or waking, and when your eyes open it will take a few moments again before you are fully orientated. It is rather more difficult to rouse oneself from a really deep trance, and it takes effort. The depth of trance also largely determines what you can do while in trance. A shallow trance is all you need to help you relax and shed any anxieties and tensions, but for more profound work, you need a deeper level of trance. A moderate trance is usually enough for pain control or for treatment programmes for various physical conditions. In order to recover deeply buried and traumatic memories, you probably would need to go into a really deep trance.

As the induction proceeds, you will feel as though you were somehow going 'deep inside yourself', which is a phrase the therapist is likely to use. At some point, when you have entered the first and shallowest stage of trance, the therapist may ask you to imagine yourself somewhere, like at the doors of a lift or at the top of a flight of stairs or of an escalator. If he suggests a lift, he will ask you to get into it and feel yourself being gently carried downwards. If the image is of stairs, he will ask you to walk down them. Images like this tend to make it easier to go into deeper levels of trance: somehow, the idea of moving downwards produces the effect of going deeper. The therapist may count from one to ten as you go down the stairs, or count backwards as the lift in which you are travelling moves down from, say, the tenth floor to the first.

At the end of this first stage, when you get out of the lift or reach the bottom of the stairs, you will feel yourself feeling really detached, and very far away from the outside world. Generally, this is a very comfortable sensation, but it can initially feel a little alarming if you are not used to being able to detach yourself in such a way. As you become more accustomed to and skilled in the use of hypnosis, you will find that this stage makes you feel extraordinarily calm and peaceful. You may feel on the first occasion that you are losing control, but if you test this out and try to take control again, for instance by making yourself come up again, you will find that actually you *are* in control and can do whatever you like. If you want to do so, you can open your eyes and be fully awake and alert again. That would mean rather a waste of time and effort, however, and it would make more sense to see what happens when you go on with what you are doing and what the therapist is suggesting.

When the therapist considers that you have reached a sufficient depth of trance (and he may ask you how you felt about that), he may ask you to imagine one or more situations or feelings, so that you can get the *feel* of what you can do in hypnosis. For instance, he may ask you to stretch out one arm, with the palm of the hand upwards, and then imagine that a large book or stone has been placed on your hand, and to imagine how this weight would feel to you. You may be surprised how vividly and realistically you will feel that weight, exactly as though a heavy object were resting on your outstretched hand. It may feel so real that you find it impossible to hold your arm up for any length of time. The strain of holding your arm up, with such a weight resting on your hand, may well become too much for your arm muscles.

A few such 'exercises' will not only help you to understand how to use images in hypnosis, but at the same time make you feel somehow better established and more secure in the hypnotic state. A therapist will use such exercises for precisely these reasons: to make it easier for you later to use the images he may suggest to enable you to achieve whatever it is that you want from treatment (relief from pain, release of tension and anxiety, to go to sleep more easily, etc.). At the same time these experiments or exercises will help you to feel comfortable and at ease in the trance.

At some point, the therapist may ask you to let yourself go backwards through time, or backwards through your own life, or in some other way to allow yourself to picture a clear image of the time and place that you agreed upon before hypnosis was begun. The purpose of this is to take you back to a specially good experience, when you were completely happy, not just so that you can remember it better, but so that the *feelings* you had at that time should come back fully. You may be quite surprised at what happens at this point, especially if you are a really good hypnotic subject. You will feel as though the room in which you were sitting a moment ago has disappeared, and that you really are, say, five years old and sitting on a donkey at the beach, having the time of your life in the sunshine. Only then will treatment begin.

In a training workshop in hypnotherapy I was conducting some time ago with a colleague, we included a session in which all workshop members were to go into a trance in a group. My colleague did the induction (that is, led the session just as a therapist does with a single individual), and as I was feeling a bit tired, I let myself go along with it, and soon was in a very pleasant trance. Then my colleague suggested that we were going down some steps to a beach. I was quite surprised when I felt myself quite unmistakably climbing down some wooden steps to a beach I had not even thought of for forty years, a beach on which I spent many happy hours as a boy, when I was playing hookey from school. I could see it, I could feel the shingle under my feet. I could even smell the seaweed. It was completely real to me, in a way that simply recalling an event usually is not, and I was very sorry when I heard my colleague's voice telling me I was now coming back to the present!

When you have spent some time in your 'special private place' (as this good event may be called), you will probably be taught how to go into trance on your own, so that you can go to your 'private place' in order to get in touch with these good feelings on your own.

At this stage of the session, the therapist may bring you back to full wakefulness and ask you to try out the method of self-hypnosis you have just been taught. He would suggest that you are returning to a waking state. When you are fully alert again, and your eyes are open, you will probably discuss the experience so far, and he may ask you to take yourself back into trance there and then.

Once back in trance, the therapist may begin on the treatment programme that was agreed between you in the preliminary discussions. However, it is often considered that simply learning how to enter the trance and discovering what you can do with it, is enough for a first session. Whether the therapist goes on to treatment at this point, or whether he leaves it to the next session depends partly in how profound, complex and difficult the treatment is likely to be.

Even if no active treatment is undertaken at the first interview, the therapist will probably suggest to you, while you are still in trance, various images and ideas for you to work on during the daily sessions of self-hypnosis he may ask you to use. This will prepare the way for the treatment to come, and train you in the techniques you will use to deal with your problem.

At the end of the session, you will again be asked to come out of the trance. This may involve walking up the stairs or being carried up by the lift or escalator, or using whatever imagery was used to help you get into trance in the first place. When your eyes are open, you will probably find yourself smiling broadly because you feel so good, and stretching comfortably because you feel so relaxed. You will feel rather as though you had woken from a really pleasant dream, and you may well wish that you were still in it. Most people I work with agree with me that hypnosis is one of the most pleasant, refreshing and comfortable experiences you can have.

Chapter 6

Can Hypnosis Help YOU?

You may well have got the impression that hypnosis can help in treatment of almost any and every condition, whether it is physical or psychological or both. The use of hypnosis for alleviating a wide variety of disorders, illnesses and difficulties has been described in earlier chapters. There are very few conditions that have not been helped in some way and to some extent by adding hypnotherapy to whatever other treatments have been applied.

It is also true that there have been some very impressive reports of the results of using hypnotic techniques in some conditions (such as cancer), that you may think would not be likely to respond to such an approach. You might therefore be tempted to ask, 'if hypnosis is so powerful and effective, why is it not used regularly, and perhaps even in preference to drugs and other physical treatments?'

One of the realities of life is that people tend to talk and write about their successes and leave their 'failures' out entirely! Reading some of the books on hypnotherapy that are to be found in the shops, you could indeed be pardoned for thinking that it is high time we gave up surgery, drugs, and just about all the armamentarium of modern medical science, and left everything to hypnosis. (Much the same reaction would be reasonable if one took some descriptions of other therapies, such as homeopathy, acupuncture and so on, completely literally!) If, however, you were to talk confidentially to a doctor or psychologist who uses hypnosis, you would hear a somewhat less optimistic account. Very few writers will admit in print that many of their patients do not seem to respond to hypnotic techniques. Most practising therapists, of whatever discipline, tend to be a little more realistic.

If you were to consult a practitioner who uses hypnosis, with a view to receiving treatment yourself, it would be rather unlikely that he would tell you if the chances of your gaining complete relief of your problem were small. For one thing, if you were doubtful about the value of treatment to yourself, the chances of it helping you would actually be reduced. Your faith in, and commitment to, the process are actually two of the most important ingredients in the treatment itself.

Yet it is important for a patient to have a realistic view of what he or she is being offered. The fact is that a proportion of people treated through hypnosis, are helped substantially, and some of these achieve complete relief from a wide range of disorders. But, and this is an important 'but', some people with the same conditions, treated in the same way and by the same methods, and perhaps even by the same therapist, do not gain any benefit at all. This includes some who find it extremely difficult or almost impossible to enter hypnosis at all. Finally, there is a third group, probably larger than either of these two groups, who gain some benefit, find some improvement or relief, but continue to suffer from their illness or pain.

There are many factors involved in determining who may benefit from this approach, and to what extent. Many of these factors are to do with the personality and lifestyle of the patient concerned. Some are to do with the circumstances in which the patient lives and the stresses that these impose on him or her. Some depend on the motivation for improvement or recovery, on commitment to the treatment, and on the degree to which the patient actually *uses* the treatment. Other factors are to do with the type, duration, and severity of the illness itself. And then, perhaps most important of all, and logically the first factor to be considered, is the 'hypnotic talent' of the patient himself.

People vary in their ability to enter hypnotic states and to use hypnotic techniques. So far, no one has been able to identify any reasons why one person is a 'good subject' and why another is not. Some writers, especially in the USA, insist that, although people do indeed vary in their ability to use hypnosis, everybody can respond to some degree. British writers tend to be more cautious (or perhaps there are differences in 'hypnotizability' between Americans and British people). Some American writers say that at least 95 per cent of their patients respond satisfactorily to hypnosis, others quote 80 per cent and so on. In Britain, most practitioners would, I think, agree with an estimate of around 65 per cent for patients responding with signficant results to hypnotherapy, while a few more gain some benefit from hypnotic relaxation. In my own practice, I find that even 65 per cent is a little on the high side, if I think of people who have gained really substantial benefit from treatment of this kind. Certainly, however, at least two out of three people get some benefit which they experience as worth while.

Age seems to have something to do with 'hypnotizability'. It is pretty generally agreed by researchers that children around the age of ten to twelve respond better to hypnosis than either younger or older people, and that response to hypnosis tends to get less as you go through the adult years. This is not universally true, in that some people go on responding very successfully to hypnosis well into the latter years, even if they have never used hypnosis in their youth. I have had patients aged seventy and more who have taken very well indeed to hypnosis and been able to use it very effectively, and, of course, I have had patients of ten and eleven years who have not responded at all!

It seems as though hypnotic talent is like any other talent: we all have it to some extent, some less, some more, and some are brilliantly gifted, while others cannot use it to any useful extent. Like any talent, however, unless you are exceptionally gifted, you have to practise to improve, and with regular and frequent practise, you will develop your talent much further.

Many of my patients are actually quite disappointed when they discover that they have to work at their own treatment.

They often hope that I would 'hypnotize them out of' their troubles, and that a few sessions with me would see the difficulty solved. Even though I explain right at the beginning that I am not going to cure them, but that I am going to teach them how to use their own abilities to manage and control their own problem or illness, they still hope for an almost instant cure. When this does not materialize, they sometimes lose hope and confidence, and never discover that they can use what they have learned to reduce their symptoms and improve the quality of their lives, if they take responsibility for putting it into effect.

Those, however, who persist with the self-hypnosis they have been taught, sometimes are surprised that what I told them at the outset is actually true. The more they use hypnosis and practise their treatment exercise, the less troubled they are by their illness, pain, or other problem. One patient, an elderly man with tension pains, heart problems, and chronic anxiety said to me once, rather ruefully, 'I've found out that the effect of hypnosis is cumulative, and I now realize I have got to keep up my practice sessions'. I sympathized with him. To get real benefit, you have to put in quite a lot of effort and time, but then, you might ask, how much is it worth to you to get better and stay better?

The only way to find out how much hypnotic talent you have is to try it out, just as the only way of assessing, say, how great a musical talent you may have is to learn to sing, or play an instrument, and to write music. There are tests that one can do to see how well someone is likely to respond to an hypnotic induction, but how well a particular person will *use* hypnosis can be assessed only by trying it out with him or her. That is often the first part of one's first hypnotherapy session.

There does not appear to be any relationship between personality and hypnotic talent. It used to be thought, many years ago only 'weak-minded' people could be hypnotized. In fact, although this idea is still quite widely believed, if anything, it is the other way around: only well-motivated and determined people, who know what they want and can apply themselves to it, respond well or get much benefit from hypnosis. People who need to feel very much in control of their lives and who are afraid to 'let go', often find hypnosis difficult at first, because it seems to them as though they are giving up control of themselves and their lives to the therapist. Sometimes such people take quite a long time, and need a lot of practice, to discover that in fact they are *gaining* control, not losing it, by going into hypnosis. There is something quite paradoxical about this: by *letting go* you find yourself *holding on better*. Zen Buddhists understand better than most westerners that relinquishing control can often release great strength. You cannot *make* yourself go into hypnosis, you can only *let* yourself go, and this can be quite frightening to anyone who has a strong need to be in control. Once, however, you have experienced it, the fear of losing control will disappear.

Trust in the therapist is also important, so people who find it hard to trust another person, especially one they do not really know, can find it very difficult to let hypnosis happen. You may feel yourself to be very vulnerable, lying back on a chair, or flat on a couch, with your eyes closed. It may feel as if a total stranger is taking over control of what you think and feel. This can be very alarming, until you discover what really happens is that you are in charge and that you direct what happens to and inside yourself. However, it is important, of course, that the therapist *is* trustworthy, and can be relied upon to act in an ethical and responsible way. After all, you are relying on him to teach you what you need to know. You depend upon him having the knowledge and skills to understand your problem and to devise the right treatment approach. Above all, you rely upon him, or her, to put his or her skills at your disposal, for your benefit, and not for some purpose or need of his or her own. You must, quite obviously, therefore, choose a therapist who has high ethical standards, as well as being appropriately qualified. This topic is dealt with in more detail in Chapter 7.

No illness, disease, or other problem exists in isolation. Falling ill, developing chronic pain, or experiencing psychological difficulties of any kind, is always related to everything else that is currently going on in your life.

Sometimes we can see this quite clearly, at other times it may be well hidden. For instance, a very large number of people who say 'I've never had a day's illness in my life', then find themselves visiting their doctor week after week when they retire. All of a sudden, they find themselves not feeling well, or developing all kinds of problems when they no longer have to go to work. Similarly, when people suffer a loss through the death of someone close and important to them, or through separation and divorce, they commonly suffer a variety of reactions. Not only do they often catch all sorts of infections or other illnesses, they also tend to have accidents, sometimes quite serious ones. This vulnerability seems to last for a period of about two years, and then they seem to recover from their susceptibility. That is, severe emotional stress takes its toll and makes itself felt in a variety of ways.

The time at which an illness strikes is often a clue which helps to identify the stress that has made the person more than usually vulnerable and so has precipitated the illness. In other instances, however, there is no clear indication such as a major event or stress, and it seems more likely that there has been a 'last straw'. Stresses may have been building up, perhaps for years, and have not been dealt with or dispersed in any way, and things have just 'got too much' for the individual, and nature takes over. The body, the mind or any aspect of the individual's total functioning may break down. His threshold of tolerance of stress has been exceeded and he can take no more.

An image that I often use in therapy with patients who have experienced such an over-load, is that of a dam or reservoir. The stresses of life are visualized as the mountain streams that run into a valley. A dam has been built across the valley to hold the water back. The dam represents the controls we exercise over ourselves: the stiff upper lip, the long-suffering, tolerant, accommodating mask we present to the world, the self-control of which we may have been so proud. Bit by bit, the water builds up behind the dam. All is well as long as there is not too much water. The dam remains sound and strong, and the sluice-gates allow any excess water to run off safely. When there is a storm in the mountains and great torrents of water rush in to the reservoir, however, the pressure may become too great for the dam, and it breaks, or at best, the water spills over the top in an uncontrolled rush. Or perhaps the dam was not well built, or has not been kept in good shape, and it cracks, and the water rushes out. Finally, it may be that the sluice-gates that normally let out a little water under careful control, have jammed or become blocked, and so do not keep the reservoir at a safe level.

This picture can be seen as a very realistic representation of what happens to people under increasing stress, especially if they experience a sudden additional stress. It can be used very effectively in hypnosis to help the individual gain control over the ways in which he deals with emotional stresses, using the idea of releasing enough of the water – the pent-up emotions – a little at a time through the sluice-gates, until the pressure on the dam is manageable again. One may even suggest that the dam is too high for safety, that it is higher than it needs to be, and should be lowered, so that the pressure never does build up to a dangerous level.

When such an emotional overload is the case, simple hypnotic relaxation as such can be a great help towards recovery, even if not directed in any way explicitly at the symptoms for which the patient seeks help. Equally, if the individual has not yet reached breaking point, but is showing increasing signs of being over-stressed, then spending time each day away from the everyday world can do a great deal to relieve the build-up of tension that is gradually destroying that person's ability to cope with life.

If, then, you feel, or your doctor is beginning to hint, that the difficulties or symptoms you are experiencing, are due to accumulating stresses that you are not facing and dealing with, then indeed, hypnotherapy might help you. Most of us are aware, I am sure, at any given moment, of some of the things that are stressing us: examinations, moving house, changing jobs, threats of redundancy, finance and so on. There are, however, also frequently areas of stress of which we may be profoundly unaware. You may well be able to find ways of dealing with those sources of stress of which you *are* aware on your own. Those others, however, of which you may be quite unconscious, require outside help. Here, especially, help from a skilled psychotherapist, with or without hypnosis, is likely to enable you to identify what is troubling you and so prepare you to deal with and resolve these underlying problems.

I sometimes feel quite disappointed when a patient, coming for a second appointment, tells me that he or she has been too busy to practise the self-hypnosis exercise I taught them at their first session. My heart sinks then, because I know that in all probability little good will come of that or of subsequent sessions. To be sure, we are all busy, but I do not believe, for instance, that the patient who 'does not have time' to practise relaxation and the treatment programme we have planned, *never* stops to have a cup of tea or coffee! It takes about ten minutes to prepare and drink a cup of something, even if you are in a hurry – and it can take less than ten minutes to have a quick dip into trance, rest and relax, and then return to your everyday life, refreshed and renewed.

No, the fact is that those who cannot find the time to practise, fail to carry out their allotted exercises because they are not sufficiently motivated. More often still, they do not *value* themselves enough to spend time on themselves and for their own well-being. There may also be considerable hidden gain in self-martyrdom. For example, a person whose life is so unsatisfying and who feels so unvalued may gain some sense of self-worth from suffering, and also from making others suffer. Some people have tied up their sense of their own identity so closely with the role of 'ill person', or 'willing martyr' that they cannot afford, quite unconsciously, to devote time and effort directed towards changing not just their health but their whole persona, the face that they present to the world and the role that they play. Anyone who does not have time or make opportunity to relax and help themselves, does not have time for their own selves.

If you want hypnosis to work for you, you have to work at it and *use* it. The therapist, as I have repeatedly said before, will not cure you. He will show you how to help and cure yourself. The hypnotic techniques will not cure you either if you do not use them at home as well as during your therapy sessions. One session a week, of which probably only a part is spent in hypnosis, will do you some good, to be sure, but whatever you gain in the session is likely to be lost in the intervening days, unless you work at it yourself.

Two points must be added to the list of factors which determine whether hypnosis could help you. First, motivation; that is, the will and desire for change is essential. It is important both for the treatment itself, and for the relief or resolution of your problem. Secondly, there must be commitment to the treatment, the techniques, and above all to the process of overcoming the problem. Without commitment no treatment process can have a chance of success.

All these factors concern primarily the person who is asking if hypnotherapy can help his illness or other problems, his attitudes, his expectations, and his hypnotic talent, and the circumstances of his life, especially any major events. The other side of the coin reflects aspects of the actual illness or problem itself. In the case of physical illnesses, disabilities, organ malfunctions and so on, and in chronic pain, the longer the condition has been present, the longer it is likely to be before you derive any major relief or improvement in response to hypnosis. This is, of course, usually true of other kinds of treatment also. Similarly, the more severe the condition, the slower the response to treatment, and the longer and more intensive treatment has to be. Often, if the symptoms are severe and have been present for some time, it is unlikely that the response to hypnosis will bring the total relief that you may have hoped for.

Let me repeat yet again – one must remember all the time that hypnosis is not a form of treatment itself. The answer as to whether it will help *you*, depends on three main questions.

1. To what extent are you hypnotizable; that is, how much

hypnotic talent do you have?

2. How much effort are you prepared to put into using hypnotic techniques, and to do so consistently?

3. Is the condition from which you suffer one which can respond to treatment of any kind?

Then there are some further questions.

4. Since whatever is troubling you is bound to be related to the way you live, are you prepared to look at your life and make the changes that would be needed to improve your condition?

5. Do you really want to get well? Or has the illness or problem become so much part of your life, and come to play so important and even valuable a part in it, that you would actually, even if unconsciously, find it difficult to give it up?

Many of these questions may be difficult or even impossible to answer at the outset. You may have to spend quite a lot of time with a therapist finding out how you really feel about all these issues. As you find out, however, so you would actually be working your way towards a more healthy approach to living.

That does not really answer the question that heads this chapter; at least, not directly. The fact is, there is much more to the question of whether *you* can be helped by hypnosis than either hypnotic techniques can successfully treat whatever troubles you, or whether you are a good hypnotic subject. The complexity of the question has perhaps become a little more apparent in this chapter.

It is simply not honest to suggest that *anyone* can be helped by hypnosis, or that *any* condition can be helped by such means. Hypnosis can be used properly only with a *person* and can be effective only if the process takes into account every aspect of that person's life.

Then, once again, even if one were to use the most sophisticated and highly developed techniques of hypnotherapy, with a person of exceptional hypnotic talent, who is highly motivated, works hard at it and is wholly committed to getting well, you would *still* need to work together on whatever other treatments were necessary. The best hypnotherapy with the best subject is still not, and must never be regarded as, a form of treatment which makes medicine, surgery, and so on, redundant. It can never be a substitute for these other therapies. Hypnosis can add to the power of other treatments, can make unpleasant and painful treatments less distressing, and can make it easier for you to make those adjustments in your life that are needed if you are to become and remain healthy.

I suppose that the only exceptions to this general rule, are those problems that are not really illnesses or psychological disorders, but with which you may need some help, as, for example, giving up smoking, nail biting, or other unwelcome, unpleasant, or unhealthy habits. Even with such simple problems as these, however, one usually needs to ask if there are hidden reasons for the fact that you have not been able to rid yourself of such a habit without help.

So the question set for this chapter is really a very complex one, despite its simple appearance. But then, we are never simple and are always complex, both in ourselves and in all the things we do. Professor Joad, in a discussion panel programme on radio many years ago was famous for beginning his answer to every question with the words, 'Well, it all depends on what you mean by...'. Whether *you* might be helped by hypnosis depends on you, what you need help with, what sort of help you need, and what you want and hope for. Magical cures are an illusion, and you will not find them in hypnosis, or anywhere else. But hypnotic techniques can be of value to most people, in one way or another.

Chapter 7

Where Can You Go For Hypnotherapy? Who Uses Hypnosis?

Although hypnosis has been around for a long time, and was approved (as long as it was used under the supervision of a doctor), by the British Medical Association more than thirty years ago, there are still relatively few people in the Health Service professions who are trained in its use, or even willing to try it. This is very different from the situation outside these professions. Every local newspaper, and many of the national papers carry advertisements inserted by people offering hypnotherapy for problems such as blushing, stammering and smoking. Hypnotherapists appear in the Yellow Pages, and usually have long strings of initials after their name, suggesting all sorts of high-powered qualifications. It does seem as though help of this kind is much more readily available outside the official services and professions than within them.

In this respect, hypnotherapy is really no different from other forms of 'alternative' therapies, and many 'natural health' centres and clinics include hypnotherapy in the list of treatments they offer. It would therefore be very easy to think that such a centre or clinic, or an individual practitioner, would be the obvious place to look for help of this kind.

There is no doubt that many of these practitioners are skilled in what they do, and that they might be helpful. However, it will already be clear from the preceding chapters, that there are substantial dangers in putting oneself in the hands of someone without a suitable and adequate background and training in other disciplines or professions.

Suppose, for example, you have had trouble with recurrent

headaches for some weeks or months. Suppose, too, that you
have become alarmed by these headaches, and by the prospect
of taking pain-killers for long periods. You decide to go to a
hypnotherapist, and, having done so, you find that you can
reduce the pain and perhaps even suppress it altogether. In
time, however, you may find that the headaches return and
they eventually become uncontrollable. You may also develop
other symptoms. Perhaps you cannot see properly, or you faint
from time to time, or some other worrying things begin to occur.
At last you go to see your doctor, and after investigation it is
found that you have something quite seriously wrong that
needs medical treatment, of which the headaches were the first
sign. By the time you get to the doctor, the condition has
become more serious still because of the lack of appropriate
attention in the early stages.

Or suppose that you have chronic indigestion and pain in
your stomach, which you think is due to tension and the stresses
of your life. Again, perhaps, you go to a hypnotherapist, who
helps you to relax and perhaps get rid of the tension to some
extent, and you feel better. One morning, you wake up to find
yourself vomiting blood, when the stomach ulcer that has been
developing perforates. At this stage of the condition you are in
serious danger.

The greatest danger from consulting and being treated by
hypnotherapists without medical qualifications and working
outside the medical field, is not that they will do you harm, but
rather that they are not equipped to make a full and thorough
diagnosis. They simply do not have the necessary training to do
this. Many may not even realize that the symptoms which they
can treat quite successfully in the short term should be taken
much more seriously right from the beginning, because they are
signals of something going wrong in aspects of your mind and
body. These practitioners lack the training, knowledge, and
experience to recognize such symptoms.

This can be true of practitioners of any and all alternative
therapies. Only those whose training has been thorough, and
who are themselves thoroughly ethical, can be relied upon to

recognize when a symptom is a signal of something more serious and therefore outside their own area of competence. Even then, they may not always recognize this reliably enough to ensure the safety of the patient by referring the patient on to the medical services.

Your first step should always be to consult your own doctor. This is true whether the problem for which you want help shows itself in physical symptoms, or whether it seems to be psychological. Let us consider several 'scenarios'.

For example, you have always been a little on the nervous side, but lately you have begun to get bouts of more severe anxiety, which occur from time to time when you are out of your home, perhaps when you go shopping. These anxiety attacks are becoming more frequent and more severe, so you decide to see your GP.

After listening to your story, and then checking you over physically, your doctor suggests that you take a tranquillizer for a few weeks and see how you get on. You do not want to take such drugs, and ask if you could have hypnotherapy instead. The doctor does not take this seriously, and tells you that hypnosis is ineffectual.

You insist politely that you would, nevertheless, like to try it, and if it proves useless then you will more happily take the medication he has suggested. You ask if he will please refer you to the local Psychological Service. He then writes to the District Psychologist, and in due course you are sent an appointment to see a Clinical Psychologist. This appointment could be at a clinic or hospital in your home area, or it might be in the GP's surgery or in a Health Centre.

The psychologist is likely to spend time with you getting to know the way you live, your relationships with your family, and your personal history, in order to make sense of the problem you are experiencing. Again you ask about hypnosis, and are told that hypnosis is rubbish or charlatanry, or not a respectable form of treatment. You point out that many Clinical Psychologists use it, that it has been approved by the BMA, that there are two societies for doctors, dentists and psychologists that provide training and support research in its use, so would he please find someone amongst his colleagues who is trained in this technique, whom you could see.

If you persist, without of course becoming unpleasant or hostile, you may very well end up seeing a qualified hypnotherapist.

There is something of a problem in this story in that doctors, psychologists and other professionals generally do not like patients trying to decide what sort of treatment they should receive. You may make yourself rather unpopular by insisting on your choice of treatment but generally, as long as you make it clear that if your chosen treatment proves unsuccessful you will accept the treatment that is being offered, you will be treated sympathetically.

There may be another outcome to this story however. When you have told your tale to your GP and he has examined you, he may then ask you to tell him about your personal history, your present way of life, your family, your work, your financial position, and all the other things that commonly put stresses on people. As the picture becomes clearer and he begins to make some sense of your anxiety attacks, the GP may himself suggest that hypnosis is the right form of treatment for you, even before you have dared to mention it! He may use hypnosis himself when he considers it appropriate. Before you leave his surgery, you will have had your first taste of the hypnotic state and will probably come away feeling rather different from how you felt when you went in.

However, it may also be that instead of treating you himself with hypnotherapy, he may arrange for you to see a Clinical Psychologist, a Psychiatrist, or perhaps another GP in the practice, who will be able to work with you in this way.

If you seek hypnosis by this route, you can be as sure as it is possible to be that you are receiving treatment in the right hands, and that if any other treatment is necessary, it will be provided. You can feel confident that any physical factors in your problem will be borne in mind, and that if in the course of treatment any further such factors begin to emerge, they will be noted and investigated.

There is another side to this, too, which you also need to bear in mind when deciding where you will go for help. In any form of treatment, whether physical or psychological, you are putting yourself in the hands of the therapist in a very special way. By asking for the therapist's help, and accepting the treatment offered, you make yourself vulnerable in several ways. You can always get up and walk out, of course, if you are asked to do something you find objectionable, or if the therapist does something which you find offensive, but by the time something like this happens, you will probably have become dependent on the therapist to some extent.

If you are being treated by a member of one of the established professions, you can be confident that the possibility of your being abused in any way is very small indeed. There are, to be sure, instances of doctors who have abused the position of trust, but compared with the number of doctors in the country and the number of patients they see, these instances are microscopically few. Doctors are subject to a very strong ethical and disciplinary code, and have been rigorously trained in the ethics of doctor–patient relationships. The same is true of all established and authentic professions. It is not true, however, of many 'fringe' practitioners.

There are quite a number of independent institutions which purport to train practitioners of hypnotherapy. These institutions, often with very impressive names and titles, are completely beyond the arm of the law. This means that the customer has no protection in law, except, of course, that anything which constitutes an assault, is subject to the same laws as any other assault. These institutions are independent in the sense that they are answerable to no one, have no legal status, and have no control over their members in the way that the General Medical Council controls and is answerable for the medical profession. They are independent also in that they themselves set their ethical standards and rules, and are not subject to any sort of public scrutiny or control. Finally, they are independent also of any public or professional scrutiny or

control of what they teach and practice. They are accountable
to no one.

In fact, more often than not, these institutions, despite their
official-sounding names, consist of a handful of individuals,
often only two or three, who have decided to set themselves up
in a lucrative business. In establishing their 'College', or
'Institute', they do so entirely without any official recognition,
and without any supervision or control of their own
'qualifications' or those they provide. Sometimes the
motivation is no doubt perfectly valid: the people involved
believe that what they have to offer is good. Sometimes,
however, the motivation is simply to get on to a 'band-wagon'
and to make money out of selling something to members of the
public that is fashionable or popular. Sadly, the aim of such
organizations is exploitation, not therapy.

Another important characteristic of these organizations is
that, very commonly, the people involved in setting them up do
not themselves hold valid clinical qualifications for the methods
they are claiming to teach and practise. Several such
organizations are run and staffed entirely by people who would
not be accepted as clinical practitioners by any of the official
societies concerned with hypnosis, since they do not hold
qualifications that are recognized in Britain. Such
qualifications as they quote in their brochures sound very
impressive, but usually mean little or nothing. They simply do
not qualify their owners for any post in, for example, the
National Health Service. It is, however, perfectly possible for
any member of the public to check up on the qualifications
claimed by both individuals and organizations. Addresses of
the two professional societies in this country, which can provide
such information, are given on p.91.

These organizations commonly advertise their services to the
general public as centres for treatment through hypnosis,
hypnotherapy and various forms of psychotherapy, and their
'graduates', who put all sorts of letters after their names,
advertise their services to the general public in the same way.
At first glance there does not seem any simple way in which the

public can discriminate between the genuine, validly qualified professionals or self-styled and unqualified practioners.

In fact, there is a very simple test you can apply: if someone advertises himself as a 'hypnotist', 'hypnotherapist' or 'psychotherapist', you can be completely certain that he is not qualified. The only professional group which allows its members to advertise is that of solicitors: all other professions forbid their members to advertise in any way. Anyone who does advertise himself, therefore, is not an accepted member of a recognized profession.

However, this test is not completely reliable as some practitioners who do not have genuine qualifications do not actually advertise – you might instead find their names on the staff lists of Natural Health Centres, or simply announced on notice boards, or on a brass plate by their house. As this is not counted as advertising, it is also quite possible that people who hold valid clinical qualifications might permit their names to appear in such settings. Your only real safeguards are: first, ask your doctor. If he does not know, you can check the qualifications claimed by the practitioner concerned by enquiring from the staff at the District Psychological Department. You can enquire from one of the two professional bodies concerned with hypnosis – the British Society of Medical and Dental Hypnosis, and the British Society of Experimental and Clinical Hypnosis. You will find the addresses of these bodies on p.91.

There is a great temptation to seek help of this kind privately. At present, and for the foreseeable future, waiting lists in all National Health Service Departments tend to be lengthy, and because of the pressure of work and the shortages of staff, the help available can be quite limited. Furthermore, there are still relatively few medical practitioners and psychologists who use hypnotic techniques, and so their waiting lists tend to be pretty full. In consequence, you may decide you wish to seek help through private practitioners. Your best, and by far your safest, plan is, as always, to ask your own doctor so that he can recommend someone whom he knows and trusts. If he cannot help you in this way, then ask one of the two societies to put you in touch with a qualified practitioner in your home area.

Always talk with your GP first. He needs to know what you are doing and what treatment you may be receiving. He is, after all, responsible for you medically. Even if he is sceptical about hypnosis – and he is much more likely to be interested, even if he does not use hypnosis himself – any ethical hypnotherapist will want to inform your doctor. He may also need to ask your doctor what he knows of your problems, what investigations have been done, what results these gave, and so on. Above all, he will need to know whether the treatment he has in mind is actually appropriate for you, and only your doctor can tell him that.

You are, of course, perfectly at liberty to consult whom you please and have whatever treatment you fancy. The law at present simply does not have any provisions for the control and supervision of any form of psychotherapy, unlike its rigorous control over the practice of medicine and surgery. In consequence, you have no protection at all, and if something goes wrong, or if you are unethically or inappropriately treated, you will have only yourself to blame. If you have a complaint, if the practitioner you consulted is not a medical practitioner or qualified member of a recognized profession, there is no outside and impartial body to whom you can complain. So, be careful. Hypnosis is a powerful tool. In the right hands, it can be tremendously helpful. In the wrong hands, it can be equally harmful.

Chapter 8

Hypnosis and Your Life

So far, the emphasis in this book has been on the use of hypnosis to deal with major problems. Various physical disorders have been mentioned, as have some more obviously psychological difficulties. A further aspect of therapeutic uses of techniques of this kind must be included, and that is the use of hypnotic techniques outside the field of disability, illness and pain. One use is the application of hypnosis to breaking habits, the other is the use of hypnotic techniques as a prophylactic, that is, as a means of guarding yourself against the development of problems, especially those that stem from stress.

Hypnosis can be used to change or treat relatively minor things. One of the most common health hazards to which we expose ourselves willingly, is smoking. We all know nowadays (even if we pretend otherwise) that smoking shortens life, exposes you to serious risk of very unpleasant diseases, and so on. Yet many people find it extremely difficult to stop smoking. Help with giving up smoking is one of the things unqualified hypnotists most commonly advertise! Hypnosis can be very helpful indeed to reduce any discomfort you may experience on giving up the habit, but it will not make you give it up. Only *your decision* to become a non-smoker can do that. However, help from a skilled therapist can support your decision and ease your path to becoming a non-smoker.

The same is true of other habitual actions, such as nail-biting, or other 'nervous habits'. For instance, if you have developed a habit of eating sweet things to excess, or always have a cake with your morning break coffee, and find it difficult to stop when you realize you are becoming over-weight, then hypnosis may help. Sometimes, just spending five minutes in a self-hypnotic trance is more pleasant and more rewarding than your chocolate bar or sticky pastry, and, after all, hypnosis is not fattening, so your problem solves itself.

Perhaps a little more seriously, hypnosis can help one guard against the build-up of tension that is all too common in modern life. I am reminded of a phrase in Matthew Arnold's poem *The Scholar Gypsy*. Arnold was inspired to write this by finding a note in a book dating from the early seventeenth century, which reported that a student at Oxford had recently left the University and joined a gypsy band to 'escape from the stress and strain of modern life'. Stress does not seem, after all, to be a twentieth-century phenomenon!

However, instead of running away to join the gypsies, a daily session of self-hypnosis, in which you spend a little time shedding the accumulation of anxieties, tension, frustration, and so on that we all build up in our daily lives, can have an enormously beneficial effect on your health and on your enjoyment of life. Such a session has very similar effects to meditation, but is rather easier for most people to learn. And, in addition, if you are in the habit of using hypnosis regularly, and have become adept at it, then you will be able to use it whenever you need. For instance, if you have to go to the dentist and have work done on your teeth, or if you get a headache, or other harmless pain, you can use hypnosis to lessen and perhaps even extinguish the pain. I find personally, that a mid-day ten minutes in trance is as good as an hour in bed, and I can then face the afternoon thoroughly refreshed.

No illness or problem, in whatever form it shows itself, exists in isolation from the rest of your life. Many people seek help or treatment for all kinds of difficulties. In effect, they ask the doctor, pyschologist or other helping agent, to cure them, to solve the problem, or to take away whatever is troubling them. Usually they will discover that they have to contribute to the healing process in ways they probably did not expect.

For instance, when you consult your doctor about a bad pain

in your lower back, which turns out to be muscular – 'lumbago' – you may expect him simply to send you off for X-rays and physiotherapy, and perhaps advise you to take things easy for a few days, while taking some pain-killing medication. You might be surprised if he asks in detail how your job is going, how you are getting on with your husband or wife, children and parents, whether you have money worries, and so on. Perhaps he might even probe more deeply into how you feel about yourself, and how you spend your free time. I went to see my GP one day because of a quite crippling pain in my left shoulder. After he had examined me physically, he asked me what sort of car I drove, and then asked where I kept my briefcase when travelling in the car. Like most people, I used to put it on the rear seat. He told me to leave it on the front passenger seat or on the floor. Within a few days, the pain faded and never came back.

Any illness, disability, pain, or whatever, ties in with what may sometimes seem quite unlikely aspects of our lives, and if the problem is to be dealt with, solved or healed, we have to do something about those facets of our lives that are connected with the problem.

Most people are not very good at looking after themselves. We put all kinds of poisons into our bodies and into our minds and store them there. The poisons accumulate and in due course affect us. The physical poisons are not the subject of this book, there are many others available on that topic. But there are also mental poisons of stress, frustration, bottled-up anger or sadness, grief, loss, fear: all the emotions and feelings which we might call 'negative': they poison us just as surely as do any toxic substances in our food and drink or in the air we breathe.

To gain real benefit from treatment of any kind for any kind of problem, we have to look very deeply and closely at our lives, and recognize those areas which may have a part to play in producing the problem. This process may involve making changes in what we do, and in how we do it. Our relationships can be poisoned by our own problems, and in turn may themselves exacerbate those problems. Our work, all too often, is a source of both conscious and unconscious stresses and inner conflicts. Disappointments, frustrations, fears and anxieties – all kinds of emotions – litter our lives and are often disregarded or are resented, and so remain unresolved. We tend to look to 'treatment', whether by drugs, 'natural remedies', or other kinds of 'alternative therapies', including hypnosis, to put right those things we are aware are going wrong, and to cure our symptoms. No treatment, however, can cure a faulty or unhealthy way of life and the effects of such a life can only be suppressed or temporarily alleviated by treatment of any kind.

Hypnosis may be able to help you very effectively to live comfortably with an untreatable disability, such as pain from an incurable and unmodifiable condition. It may help you to mobilize the natural healing powers of your body and mind to bring them to bear on an illness or problem. Unless you change what has caused the problem, however, you are on a losing streak. Only if you begin to look after yourself fully, and change unhealthy and illness-producing aspects of your way of life, can hypnosis or any other therapeutic technique help get you back on the path to real health.

To achieve this, however, hypnotic techniques can be helpful. With the help of a skilled therapist, you may be able to uncover the stresses and conflicts that make you suffer. Then you can begin to tackle them. This is not something you will do in one or two sessions. It is a major task, to which you must be fully committed if you are to derive the best from it. It is also a task which will involve taking a long, hard look at your life, and changing a great deal of what, up to now, you may have taken for granted. The more serious and long-standing the problem, the longer, and probably harder, that process is likely to be.

Hypnosis is a powerful process, and can be very helpful in the many ways I have described. However, it can be misused, not only out of ignorance, lack of skill, or carelessness, but also to exploit the susceptible. It can also be misused on oneself. Just as an untrained therapist may misdiagnose your condition, you may do the same yourself.

If, for example, you have pain, that pain is an indication of something wrong somewhere in your whole being. It may be primarily physical, it may be primarily mental or emotional, or it may just be that you have been over-doing things and are stressed and over-tired. If you use self-hypnotic techniques to make yourself unaware of the pain, you could be storing up trouble for yourself by postponing the time when you seek professional help. You should not, therefore, use self-hypnosis in the same way that some people use aspirin: as a treatment for any pain or discomfort as soon as it appears. You must first be sure that whatever is wrong is only tiredness or something equally natural, and not potentially dangerous. And even then, perhaps you should look at the *reasons why* you have developed this pain, and perhaps think about making changes in some aspects of your life that will make it more healthy, and therefore reduce the likelihood of a reason for pain or other physical sign of distress occurring.

Hypnosis, then, can be a valuable technique in providing treatment for a wide range of troubles and disorders. In addition, it can be a very valuable aid to improving the quality of your life. It is not magical, mysterious, occult, or even strange, but something that occurs in the lives of most people naturally and spontaneously. It has been used by mankind throughout recorded history, and probably even well before man started leaving records of his beliefs and actions. From time to time in its history, it has unfortunately fallen into disrepute and even become the province of charlatanry and deceit. Sometimes, too, it has been treated merely as an entertainment. During the course of this century, however, it has developed into a much better understood and more scientific technique, and is now becoming increasingly an integral part of the healing arts. It is a powerful tool, and should not be used lightly, carelessly, or without proper training and professional skills. Used with respect and care, however, it may produce beneficial and healing results.

Afterword

I hope that this account of hypnosis and hypnotherapy has cleared away some of the common misunderstandings that exist around the subject. This book has necessarily been brief, and the account lacking, perhaps, in detail. There is now a vast number of books on the subject, written primarily for the practitioner or for those engaged in research. Most of these are rather technical, and not always easy to read. If you would like to read more deeply on the subject, I would recommend *Hypnosis: its Nature and Therapeutic Uses* by H. B. Gibson, published by Peter Owen, London, in 1977.

Useful Addresses

The British Society of Medical and Dental Hypnosis
Secretary: Ms M. Samuels,
42, Links Road,
Ashtead,
Surrey.

The British Society of Experimental and Clinical Hypnosis
Secretary: Dr M. Heap,
Department of Psychology,
Middlewood Hospital,
Sheffield.

Overseas

Australia:

The Australian Society for Hypnosis
Secretary: Mrs Cathryn Gow
53, Stewart Road
Ashgrove
Queensland 4060

USA:

The Society for Clinical and Experimental Hypnosis
Secretary: Dr G. Gail Gardner
University of Colorado Medical Centre
Colorado

Index